# Medical Evidence
# A Handbook for Doctors

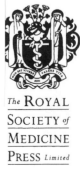

*The* ROYAL
SOCIETY *of*
MEDICINE
PRESS Limited

© 2001 Royal Society of Medicine Press Ltd.
1 Wimpole Street, London W1G 0AE, UK
207 Westminster Road, Lake Forest, IL, 60045, USA
www.rsmpress.co.uk

**British Library Cataloguing in Publication Data**
A catalogue record for this book is available from the British Library

ISBN: 1-85315-387-7

Phototypeset by Phoenix Photosetting, Chatham, Kent

Printed in Great Britain by Bell and Bain Ltd, Glasgow

# ▶ Preface

Medical evidence in criminal and civil proceedings, in courts and in tribunals of all kinds, is the subject of this work. Medicine and the law have long had an intimate and sometimes tense relationship. Doctors, like all other citizens, may sometimes fall foul of the law; in that respect they are in no sense special, save only that there are certain 'medical crimes' which only healthcare professionals have the opportunity to commit.

As professional and expert witnesses, doctors are able to assist the court by applying their special knowledge in the forensic context. It is sometimes assumed that any doctor, properly trained in his art, can function as a competent professional or expert witness. It is the experience of those of us who have tried it, however, that it isn't quite as simple as that. Lawyers 'play by different rules' than doctors; they seek to win their case, not to achieve consensus. It is important for doctors who give evidence in court to understand the differences in approach and to understand 'where the lawyer is coming from'. This book sets out to assist those who have ambitions to become professional or expert witnesses (and indeed those doctors who are asked to give evidence in court sporadically – as will happen with most doctors at some point in their career) to understand the basic requirements.

In his inaugural lecture to the new Provosts Lecture Series at University College on 17 January 2001, the Lord Chief Justice, Lord Woolf, expressed the view that the court had until recently treated the medial profession with excessive deference. He went on to say that he thought the position was changing, attributing the change to a number of factors – including the increasing frequency of litigation against healthcare professionals, the growth in judicial review, public expectations of the profession's responsibilities and the denting of the 'automatic presumption of beneficence' attributed previously to doctors and destroyed recently by public scandal. He pointed out that the number of complaints to the General Medical Council had risen from 3000 last year to a predicted 4300 in the current year. He could well have gone on to mention that in 1975 there were only 500 recorded NHS claims for negligence, whereas in 1992 there were 6000, and the projected cost of these claims in 2001 is £500 million, with total costs of outstanding claims estimated at about £2 billion.

With increasing numbers of cases in civil and criminal courts and before disciplinary tribunals, there is an ever increasing need for medical evidence and, perhaps more importantly, for the quality of that evidence to be improved. Both in the criminal and civil field there have been well-publicized recent examples of medical witnesses failing, at least in the view of the judiciary, to provide accurate independent and unbiased testimony to the courts.

In his previous role as Master of the Rolls (the head of the civil division of the Court of Appeal), Lord Woolf recommended reforms of civil justice, subsequently enshrined in the Civil Procedure Rules (1998), which came into effect on 26 April 1999. Particularly in the area of expert evidence (Part 35), these rules have had a significant effect upon the role and duties of the expert. Lord Justice Auld's review of the criminal procedure, currently under way, is likely to have a similar effect.

A further engine for change is the recent creation of the Council for the Registration of Forensic Practitioners, a body that currently assesses and accredits some forensic experts in the criminal courts and has ambitions to expand its activities to encompass all expert evidence given in those courts, and to begin to influence experts in the civil courts.

When the Civil Procedure Rules were introduced, it was widely supposed that because they set out to limit the extent of expert evidence and the cost of that evidence, there would be a diminution in the expert witness industry. Andrew Horrocks (litigation partner at Barlow Lyde and Gilbert), writing in *The Times* on 2 May 2000, commented:

> The reforms have heralded a change on experts. At our recent Woolf seminar, Mr Justice Lightman said experts were already an 'expensive luxury' and their evidence often irrelevant. In our view they will become less common.

Experience at the Expert Witness Institute suggests wide variation according to the profession of the expert; whilst work seems to have contracted for some (for example, employment consultants have been particularly badly affected), in medicine the situation appears to be different. Expensive luxury or not, it is difficult to see how the courts could manage without clinical experts in personal injury cases and there seems to be little diminution in demand. In addition to their old responsibilities of writing reports, commenting and advising on pleadings, attending conference with counsel and appearing at trial, the expert is now frequently required to assist in the drafting of questions to the opposing experts (within 28 days of the service of reports) and in turn answering questions from the other party. Experts are frequently required to assist in the planning of experts' discussions and subsequently to take part in those discussions, all at very short notice. In fact, the complaint – particularly from claimant solicitors in clinical negligence litigation – is that there are simply not enough experts available to respond within the court timetables. The need is for *more* experts, not fewer. More experts with more time are required, and those experts need education and training.

There is increasing need for medical evidence in other courts and tribunals. The quality of expert evidence is important if the needs of justice are to be served properly. Poor-quality evidence leads to injustices. Legal aspects of medical practice are not well taught in the UK, whether at undergraduate or postgraduate level. Giving medical evidence in various courts and tribunals can be a stimulating challenge and is essential to the proper administration of justice. The opportunity exists for doctors of maturity and experience from all specialities to become professional or expert witnesses; the purpose of this book is to provide an introduction, basic instruction and a signpost to further learning. The contributors of the various chapters are experienced practitioners in their respective fields.

*Roger Clements*
*March 2001*

# ▶ Contents

# ▶ List of Contributors

**John Bradley** FRCP FRCPsych
*Medical Member: Mental Health Review Tribunal*

**Roger V Clements** FRCS FRCOG
*Editor: Clinical Risk; Governor: Expert Witness Institute*
111 Harley Street, London W1G 6AW, UK

**Denis D'Auria** MA, LLM, MD, DIH, CBiol MIBiol, FFOM
*Consultant Occupational Physician and Director, Occupational Health Services, Barts and the London NHS Trust; Director, Legge-Hunter Centre; Honorary Senior Lecturer in Occupational Medicine, St Bartholomew's and the Royal London School of Medicine and Dentistry*
*Legge Hunter Centre, Occupational Health Services, St Bartholomew's Hospital, West Smithfield, London EC1A 7BE, UK*

**Neville Davis** *MBE* FRCGP FFOM
*Senior Forensic Medical Examiner, Metropolitan Police; Hon. Sec. Education and Training Programme, Expert Witness Institute; Hon. Med. Sec. Medico-Legal Society*
*Redroofs, Windmill Lane, Arkley, Herts EN5 3HX, UK*

**Roy N Palmer** LLB MB BS DObstRCOG, Barrister-at-Law
*Medico-Legal Consultant; Deputy Coroner; Governor: Expert Witness Institute; Secretary and Medical Director of the Medical Protection Society 1989–1998*
*Southwark Coroner's Court, Tennis Street, London SE1 1YD, UK*

**Raina Patel** MB ChB MRCGP DRCOG DMJ
*Romiley Health Centre, Chichester Road, Romiley, Stockport, Cheshire SK6 4QR, UK*

# ▶ Table of Cases

Entries are listed thus: **Chapter** (page); *reference number*

# ▶ Table of Statutes

Entries are listed as: **Chapter** (page on which each Act is mentioned)

# ▶1

# General Principles

## Introduction

Medical evidence may be written or oral, and thus this chapter both includes the preparation of written reports and appearances in court to give oral evidence. Most doctors will be called upon to prepare a report for medico-legal purposes or to give evidence in court at some stage in their careers. If a few basic principles are understood clearly, giving evidence can be an interesting diversion and a stimulating experience. However, equally it can be a harrowing and miserable experience if the basic rules are ignored.

Be aware of the differences between evidence of *fact* and evidence of *opinion*. The fact that you are a doctor does not mean that evidence you give is expert evidence. You may simply be asked to provide factual evidence about a patient, such as a description of a patient's condition and the treatment that you provided. An expert opinion usually will involve an interpretation of facts (often facts ascertained by other practitioners, by way of a review of medical records), such as an evaluation of a prognosis or of the standard of care provided. Of course, some medico-legal reports will contain a mixture of fact and opinion, but it is always important to make the distinction (if only in your own mind) between the two.

Be aware, too, of the difference between 'best' evidence (ie matters witnessed by your own senses) and 'hearsay' evidence (eg Angela told me that Brenda told Catherine she had..., and so on).

## Duty of care

It is important to be clear about those to whom you owe a duty of care when preparing medical evidence. The duty is owed to the person who commissions the evidence.

If you are asked to prepare a report on a patient whose clinical care you have been responsible for and you are asked to examine and report upon that patient, it will be important to make clear to the patient that, in the context of the exercise, you are not his/her doctor but that you must provide an unbiased and objective report (with the patient's consent) to whomever has commissioned it. There is scope for confusion and misunderstanding if the patient thinks that he is attending another clinical consultation with 'his' doctor and fails to understand the purpose of the assessment. Again, your duty of care in the preparation of the medical evidence is owed to those who commissioned the report.

If you have never been responsible for the clinical care of the individual and you are asked to prepare a report that includes the results of a clinical examination, you owe a duty of care to the individual 'patient' not to harm him in the course of your examination. Beyond that, however, you do not owe the individual a duty of care; your duty of care for the content of your report is owed to the person or organization which commissioned it. This is particularly relevant in the context of occupational health assessments and assessments of insurance claims. A doctor engaged by an employer to advise on the suitability of prospective employees for employment does not owe a duty of care to an applicant who completes a medical questionnaire. The Court of Appeal has held[1] that there is no special relationship between a doctor and a job applicant such as to give rise to a duty of care.

## Confidentiality

Doctors will receive requests for information from a variety of sources. These include lawyers, employers, social service departments and insurance companies. It is important first to ensure that you have the consent of the individual about whom you are asked to prepare a report. That individual must agree that you may provide details about him/her to the person who has requested it. If you have not been provided with the consent of the individual (which only exceptionally may be inferred, such as when the request comes from the person's own legal adviser), you must insist upon having it before you submit your report.

It would be a breach of confidentiality for you to provide to others information that you have gained in the course of your professional duties without the consent of the individual about whom the report is to be prepared. Guidance on confidentiality is readily available from the General Medical Council (GMC),[2] from the medical protection and defence organizations (Medical Protection Society [MPS], Medical Defence Union [MDU], and Medical and Dental Defence Union of Scotland [MDDUS]) and from the British Medical Association (BMA).

If a patient personally, or that patient's lawyer, asks you to prepare a report, consent is implicit in the request. For all other requests for information about a patient, the doctor must ensure that s/he has been provided with the requisite consent. It is very important, however, to avoid confusion between roles in the preparation of a medico-legal report. The report is prepared for the benefit of the client on the instructions of the client or the client's legal adviser; it is not open to the doctor to assume a clinical or therapeutic relationship and to disclose copies of the medico-legal report to other doctors who have clinical responsibility for the care of the patient unless and until the patient has given express consent for that to occur.

Copies of medical reports should not be given voluntarily to any third party, least of all the other parties in the litigation, without the consent of the person who commissioned them. It is best to refer requests for copies to the legal adviser to whom the report was addressed.

*Legal professional privilege* may also attach to your report. A report commissioned by a lawyer on behalf of a client may be legally privileged, so that no one else has any right to see it and you may be protected from any proceedings for defamation for what you state in such a report. Waiver of privilege is a matter for the client (or his lawyer) who commissioned the report.

However, there may be circumstances where you, as a doctor, consider that you have an ethical duty to disclose the contents of your report even though the lawyer and his client refuse to allow you to do so. One such case was that of *W v Egdell*,[3] in which a psychiatrist was asked to assess and report upon a dangerous patient who was seeking discharge from compulsory detention under an order of the Mental Health Act 1983. The psychiatrist did not believe that the patient was fit for release but the patient and his lawyers wanted the report to remain confidential. The psychiatrist was so concerned that he disclosed the report, without consent, to those responsible for the care of the patient. The Court of Appeal upheld the psychiatrist's decision and dismissed the claim by the patient for breach of confidentiality, holding that the psychiatrist had acted responsibly, in the public interest. Such cases are rare, however, and doctors would do well to seek medico-legal advice when faced with one.

## Immunity from legal action

Advocates used to enjoy immunity from legal action for their professional work in court (albeit that immunity from litigation for their advice and opinions was withdrawn some years ago). Witnesses, whether expert or otherwise, have also enjoyed immunity from litigation for what they said in court. The rationale was that they had to feel free and unfettered by concerns that they might be sued for their trouble in assisting the court if justice was to be done properly.

In a recent decision of the House of Lords, however, advocates lost their immunity from litigation for their professional work in court, both in civil and in criminal matters.[4] The decision of their lordships was unanimous insofar as civil cases are concerned but was reached only by a majority of a seven-man House insofar as criminal cases is concerned. The decision also reversed previous decisions of the House of Lords that dealt with the immunity of advocates.

The case dealt only with immunity for advocates and did not deal with evidence from experts and other witnesses, but there would appear to be a possibility that experts who are paid to give their opinions in court (if not other witnesses of fact) might also lose their immunity for what they say in evidence. The point is not entirely clear at the time of writing, but those who agree to act as experts might wish to bear it in mind.

## Access to Medical Reports Act 1998

Under the provisions of the Access to Medical Reports Act 1988, individuals about whom reports are prepared for employment or insurance purposes have certain statutory rights to see the report and to comment upon it before the report is passed to the person or body that asked for it. The provisions of the Act apply to medical reports prepared for employment or insurance purposes by any doctor who is or has been responsible for the clinical care of the individual – and thus do not apply to doctors who have never at any time been responsible for clinical care.

A duty is imposed upon insurance companies and employers to notify the individual about whom the report is requested of his rights, and to obtain his consent before an approach is made to the doctor for a report. The individual has a right to refuse consent and to see the medical report, and to request amendments to be made before it is dispatched to the commissioning organization. The organization, in approaching the doctor, must notify him if the patient has expressed a wish to see the report and the doctor then must not dispatch the report unless the patient has seen it or has failed to make arrangements to see it within 21 days. The individual has some rights to request corrections of errors. The Act also requires the doctor to retain copies of medical reports for six months and to allow the individual access to them upon request. There are some exceptions to the provisions of the Act, particularly in circumstances where the doctor believes that disclosure of the report, or part of it, might cause serious harm to the mental or physical welfare of the individual or other persons.

More detailed guidance on the operation of the Act is available from, *inter alia,* medical protection and defence organizations (eg MPS, MDU and MDDUS) and from the BMA.

# Disclosure of expert reports

Doctors who provide expert medical advice for the defence in criminal cases have, since 1987, been required to prepare the reports in a form in which they can be disclosed to the prosecution. Further changes to the rules may arise after the publication of the report by Lord Justice Auld into the practices, procedures and rules of evidence in criminal courts at every level currently (as of December 2000) underway.

In civil cases, the Civil Procedure Rules[5] – introduced as a consequence of the reforms recommended by Lord Woolf in his Report *Access to Justice*[6] and operative since April 1999 – have radically altered the way in which expert evidence is dealt with.

A comparable, comprehensive review of the operation of criminal law and procedure is currently being undertaken under the chairmanship of Lord Justice Auld. When published, it, like the Woolf proposals, is likely to lead to profound changes in the criminal justice system in England and Wales. These topics will be dealt with in the relevant chapters of the book.

# What is required?

You must be clear that you understand what is wanted before you prepare a report or give oral evidence. Not all requests for information are clear – and lawyers' requests are no exception. Your report must be directed to the purpose for which it was requested, and if that is unclear you should seek clarification. Thus, what is required depends on the circumstances.

Does the person who asked for the report want a report on the facts, such as a narrative account, in chronological order, of a patient's management and progress following an illness or accident? Or is the request for an opinion, such as whether the patient may be expected to make a full recovery following an accident or suffer later complications, and when s/he will be fit to return to work? Or is the request for an expert opinion on the management of the clinical care – whether those responsible for looking after the patient were negligent?

If you are to act as an expert witness, be sure to understand the relevant test. The rules of evidence in English law differ between criminal and civil cases. The standard of proof in a criminal case is the higher one of 'beyond reasonable doubt' (also known as 'satisfied so that you are sure'), whereas the standard in civil cases is on the 'balance of probabilities' ('more likely than not'). Doctors do not need to know the details of the rules of evidence but should know that differences exist.

Quite apart from the usual criminal and civil courts (such as the magistrates' courts, county courts, the Crown Court and High Court), there are many other courts and tribunals at which you might be asked to give evidence. Examples include (but the list is certainly not exhaustive, nor is it intended to be) Coroners' Courts (sheriffs' courts in Scotland), mental health review tribunals, industrial tribunals, courts martial and disciplinary tribunals (eg the GMC, GDC, UKCC, Council for Professions Supplementary to Medicine, etc.). Each tribunal tends to have its own rules of evidence and procedure.

Lawyers (and others who instruct doctors) should provide the necessary guidance. If they fail to do so, you should have no hesitation in asking for guidance and to know what is expected of you. For example, your report in a criminal case, especially one requested by the prosecution, might need to be set out in a special form. You might not be examined on your report at trial, but the report will have been made available to the defence, and the counsel for each 'side' may well have formulated their line of questions on the basis of what was in the report, albeit that the line the questions take at trial will very much depend on oral evidence given in the course of the trial. On the other hand, since recent reforms in civil cases in England and Wales, it is now most unusual for an expert witness to be examined 'in-chief' on the report; instead, everyone will have read the report before the trial starts and the experts will go straight in to a rigorous cross-examination on what they wrote.

So, take great care to understand the nature of the case and what is expected of you if you wish to avoid embarrassments in court. Make sure that the lawyers who commission your evidence explain matters to your complete satisfaction.

## Do I get a fee?

A question frequently posed by doctors who are called to give evidence is whether they will get a fee and, if so, how much it will be. There is no simple answer. If the evidence is simply evidence of fact in a criminal case and the doctor is called as a citizen who happened to witness certain events rather than in a professional capacity, s/he will be treated no differently from any other comparable witness.

If the doctor is called as a professional witness of fact (eg to recount his treatment of a patient), a fee may well be payable, but it may be a disappointingly small one. Fees for witnesses in criminal cases and in coroners' courts tend to be set by statutory authority and there will be little or no scope to argue. If the doctor is called as a true expert witness, a more substantive fee may be paid but it will vary considerably. In criminal cases, the fee may be set by some statutory authority and be non-negotiable. In civil cases, there may be more scope to negotiate a fee but if the case is one supported by public funds (eg a legally aided case), the fee offered might be constrained by what the legal aid authority is prepared to pay, or the amount allowed by the court official who decides on what fees are appropriate. It is not possible in this book to set out the various fees in detail, but doctors who give medical evidence should be aware of the variability in fees payable and seek advice from, for example, the BMA.

## Consequences of giving evidence

It is important to take great care in the preparation of medical evidence, whether in a written report or orally, in court. Just as much care should be taken as in any other professional work performed by a doctor. In a criminal case, poor-quality evidence may lead to an inappropriate criminal conviction and all that it entails – possible loss of liberty or fine, possible loss of job or office, social stigmatization and opprobrium. It may also lead to an undeserved acquittal with all the implications for the victims of the crime.

In a civil matter, poor-quality evidence may lead to a claim being pursued that is doomed to failure, leading to false hopes and expectations in one party and great stress and inconvenience to the other, not to mention the waste of time and costs for all concerned. Poor evidence may, conversely, mean that a deserving claimant is dissuaded from pursuing a meritorious claim.

## You may be liable to medico-legal consequences

It is as possible to be found negligent for the preparation of a medical report as for the performance of clinical work if the standard falls below that which is reasonably to be expected of those who hold themselves out as being competent to give medico-legal evidence. If you produce a sub-standard report upon which reliance is placed and an individual suffers loss as a consequence, you may be sued for damages. Indeed, if you breach confidentiality in the preparation of a report you also may have to answer to the Professional Conduct Committee of the GMC.

In a very recent case[7] (as yet unreported and understood at proof [March 2001] to be under appeal), damages were awarded for injury to feelings caused by a doctor's breach of confidence. A psychiatrist was asked to prepare a medico-legal report for a claimant's solicitors in connection with an unfair dismissal claim. The psychiatrist sent copies of the medico-legal report, without the patient's consent, to the patient's GP and to another consultant psychiatrist.

The courts, as well as the GMC, have a role in cases of alleged breach of confidence.

Publications of the medical protection and defence organizations (see past annual reports and issues of their respective journals) contain examples of claims that have arisen from negligently prepared reports. Such claims may arise because the doctor who prepared them was insufficiently thorough – for example, by missing important information discernible from medical records or by failing to review all relevant features.

## Example 1

A doctor prepared a report on the condition and prognosis for a man who had been injured in an accident. The doctor reviewed the notes but relied on someone else's written interpretation of the radiographic findings. He gave a prognosis that there would be no long-term sequelae from the injuries and the claim was settled on that basis for a modest sum. Subsequently, it transpired that the injuries had included a fracture through the articular surface of the knee joint with the consequent risk that arthritis might develop later. Had that been stated at the time of the report, the claim would have attracted much greater compensation. The report was judged to have been prepared negligently and the doctor's protection organization had to settle a claim for damages and costs to reflect the difference between the damages the patient actually recovered and what he would have recovered had the full facts and prognosis been known at the time.

## Example 2

A doctor prepared a report about a patient who had suffered a head injury in an accident. No mention was made of the possibility of the later onset of fits and the claim was settled. The patient later developed fits, which were attributed to the original injury. A claim was made against the doctor for his failure to mention the possibility of the later onset of fits; had he done so, the claim would have attracted significantly higher compensation.

## Example 3

A psychiatrist was asked by the lawyer for one party to a divorce to prepare a report. In the report, he also included details about the other party without that party's consent. A complaint was made to the GMC and the psychiatrist was reprimanded for a breach of confidentiality.

## Guidance for experts

Experts are those who the courts recognize as being competent to express an opinion, usually on the basis of facts established by other witnesses but often also on the basis of a medico-legal assessment of a patient which they, themselves, make. Further guidance on how to deal with evidence in civil and criminal matters is set out in the relevant chapters later in this book.

With the increasing volume of litigation, both civil and criminal, there are insufficient experts available with the time and inclination to devote to expert work. Many lawyers, who may experience considerable difficulty in finding experts willing to act, will approach doctors with a request to provide an opinion. The invitation may seem flattering and the task interesting and lucrative. However, only agree to act if you have the appropriate skills, knowledge, expertise and time (or you are prepared to acquire them).

If you intend to act as an expert witness you must take steps to learn how to do so correctly. There are now organizations that exist to provide guidance for experts, including courses and seminars. They include the Academy of Experts and the Expert Witness Institute (EWI).[8] Those who act regularly as experts would be well advised to join such an organization and perhaps also the Section of Clinical Forensic and Legal Medicine of the Royal Society of Medicine[9] and the Medico-Legal Society.[10]

## It's serious

In both criminal and civil cases, lawyers and the courts place great weight and reliance on the statements and opinions of experts. Agreeing to act as an expert is an onerous obligation; it is not to be undertaken lightly or unwisely. A case may succeed or fail on the basis of the medical evidence given and thus individuals may be imprisoned or fined or required to pay compensation as a consequence. The professional and lay press in recent years has contained several examples of miscarriages of justice as a result of discredited forensic evidence.

## Council for the Registration of Forensic Practitioners (CRFP)

In response to these miscarriages of justice arising from poor forensic scientific evidence, and to promote public confidence in forensic practice in the UK, a new independent regulatory body has been created. It is the Council for Registration of Forensic Practitioners (CRFP) based at Burlington House,

Piccadilly, London. It has a website (www.crfp.org.uk) containing information about its constitution and functions.

The intention is to create a register of forensic practitioners who are, and remain, competent to practise in the forensic professions. Registration will be voluntary, at least in the first instance, but the stated desire of CRFP is for 'providers and users of forensic services to come to see the register as a definitive indicator of competence'. Registration is intended to define, sustain and raise standards. The CRFP has drawn up a code of conduct: *Good Practice for Forensic Practitioners*. Every applicant for registration will be required to agree to abide by the code. CRFP will periodically reassess practitioners to ensure continuing competence. It will also have an investigatory and disciplinary function, dealing with complaints about a forensic practitioner's professional conduct, performance or state of health. There will be a charge for registration.

## What to say and how to say it

What you say depends on what you are asked (see above: 'What is required?'). Get clear in your own mind whether you are being asked for a factual report or an opinion, or both. If a factual report, read the request carefully and answer it; as with 'finals', answer the question asked and not the one you would like it to have been. If a solicitor wants a factual report about injuries sustained by his client in an accident, he will not thank you for a lengthy report detailing the full history of a chronic attender at the surgery with bulky medical records. If in any doubt about what is wanted, seek clarification before you prepare the report.

If an expert opinion is requested, be sure that you understand the points in issue. If you don't, probably because the lawyer has not made them clear, insist upon them being explained. It is often helpful for the lawyer to set out the issues in the form of a series of questions to which you are asked to respond. If the matter is outside your field of expertise, do not hesitate to say so; you will be thanked for conceding your ignorance so that the lawyer can look elsewhere for answers, but you will *not* be thanked and might even be sued for negligence if you venture an opinion which is beyond your expertise and which subsequently turns out to be wrong. Much time and costs are wasted by so-called experts straying outside their brief or specialist knowledge. And *never* parade as fact that which is mere opinion.

The issues in a case may, for example, arise from the following: (1) whether or not there was a failure to deliver a reasonable standard of care; (2) whether such a failure in the standard of care was actually causative of all the harm which allegedly flowed from the breach; or (3) what are the prospects for a recovery – when will it occur, will it be complete and are there any long-term risks? In many cases, the issue may be the difference (if any) in prognosis had care been optimal from what it is as a result of negligent care. Issue (1) is an issue of liability – was the standard of care what it should have been? Issues (2) and (3) concern quantum (ie how much the claim is worth).

Unless you are absolutely clear about the issues in the case, your report might not properly address them and may be of scant assistance to the lawyers or to the court.

Written reports should be clear and unambiguous. Try to avoid abbreviations and jargon; or at least define them when you first use them. Do not assume knowledge on anyone's part. The issues might seem clear to you because of your training and experience but they will not necessarily be clear or be understood by 'lay' persons. Set out the facts in a clear, logical, concise manner. Analyse the facts and interpret them. Address the issues raised in the lawyer's request. Do not hesitate to raise additional issues in your report if the lawyer has not thought of them but you believe them to be relevant and important. This is especially the case in civil cases where, since the Civil Procedure Rules (CPR) came into force in 1999, you have an over-riding responsibility to the court and not to the lawyer or client. This is explained more fully in the relevant chapter, later in this book.

## Appearing in court

It is almost inevitable that, as a doctor, you will have to give evidence in court sooner or later. Try to enjoy it – or at least to accept it as an interesting challenge. However, the reality is far different from how it is made to appear in films and on television. Court proceedings are, for the most part, slow and rather boring – not unlike 'watching paint dry'. Only very rarely is there drama and a 'rise in temperature'.

Accept the fact that you will feel you are 'being messed around'. There will be broken fixtures, revised dates for appearances, long waits (often in draughty corridors) and a dismal absence of facilities such as writing tables, telephones and decent catering. Despite the firm belief of many doctors to the contrary, lawyers and judges usually will try to accommodate their busy schedules but there may be many competing interests and demands on a range of witnesses such that one individual's preferences simply cannot be accommodated. The estimated duration of the length of time a witness will be 'in the box' may be misjudged, so that other witnesses may be called on earlier or, more usually, will have a longer wait than anticipated.

Courts work on the same principle as hospital outpatient clinics and GPs' surgeries – that is, that the great man (in this case, the trial judge) must never be kept waiting, no matter how many other people are. Those who regularly give evidence in courts of law recognize this and adjust to it, dealing with other work as best they can whilst waiting to give their evidence. Those who seldom give evidence and who have busy clinical commitments usually find the delays and inconveniences a major irritation – but noisome protest is unhelpful and it is better to be resigned in advance and to take suitable reading material to while away the waits.

When you are called to give your evidence, it helps to remember a few basic rules, as set out below.

### ► Stand up

Attendance at court should be a serious matter. Medical evidence often involves cases of death or serious personal injury. Your demeanour and dress should be suitable to the occasion. You should look professional – appearing in casual clothes may seem insulting and may detract from the weight that will be attached to what you have to say in evidence.

### ► Speak up

Your evidence should be given audibly and clearly. Court architecture and acoustics are not always conducive to audibility – the Victorians apparently were more concerned with grandeur and making a suitable impression on the citizenry, and many English courts are of that era. Do not mumble; make sure that you can be heard and understood by counsel, judge and jury. Try to avoid jargon, or at least explain it carefully.

### ► Shut up

Conventionally, evidence takes the form of questions and answers. Listen carefully to the question posed by counsel or the judge. Think about what you wish to say by way of an answer before you allow words to issue forth from your mouth. If you have not understood the question, ask for it to be repeated or clarified. Give your answer as accurately and concisely as possible – and then stay silent. Do not give a diatribe or lecture. Answer what is asked and not what you would like the question to have been.

A garrulous witness is a gift to an astute counsel, who will be pleased to allow the witness 'enough rope to hang himself'. If you have not answered clearly or adequately, be assured that counsel or the judge will pose another question. However, you should avoid being 'browbeaten' or intimidated into giving a 'yes' or 'no' answer if that is impossible. If a question can only be answered by a qualified answer or by some additional explanation, you must give it – because you owe a duty to the court and you have taken an oath or affirmation to tell not only the truth but 'the whole truth and nothing but the truth'.

► **Watch the judge's pen**

Do watch the judge's pen (or laptop). He will almost certainly be making notes even though there may be a stenographer or tape recording in court. Adjust the speed of your evidence accordingly. There may be silences in court; this is usually because the counsel are waiting politely for the judge to make his notes before moving on to the next question – or sometimes because counsel is thinking of the next question to ask. An inexperienced witness may think that everyone is waiting for him to say something further and will start to fill the silences with words. Avoid that temptation.

► **Stick to what you know and be prepared to admit what you *don't* know**

► **You will be respected for being frank and honest**

► **You will have an unhappy time if you dissemble or are discovered to be untruthful**

If you are asked a question of fact, stick to the facts. Do not guess or embellish; do not speculate or hypothesize. If you are giving opinion evidence, be sure to keep within your area of knowledge and expertise. Once you are shown, on cross-examination, to be wrong on one point, you make it easy for counsel to start to insinuate that no one in court can rely on anything else you have stated. If you don't know the answer, or it is outwith your specialist field, do not hesitate to say so.

You will be respected for being frank and honest and for being seen to be trying to assist the court with your answers. Do not trespass beyond the limits of your knowledge and expertise and be resolute in resisting any temptation from counsel or the judge to do so. Do not, however, be inflexible, rigid or perverse in adhering to your opinion if new facts emerge which render it no longer tenable. Be prepared to concede a point if it is sound and well made. However, do not concede a point if you cannot honestly and responsibly agree to do so – a witness who too readily departs from his previous written opinion can be a menace and can waste a great deal of time and costs.

► **Know the difference between fact and opinion** (see above)

► **Do not present as fact that which is opinion** (see above)

► **Do not take sides or appear to be partisan**

It is most important for those who give evidence to understand that they are there to assist the court to do justice between the parties in the case. The lawyers are paid to act as advocates of the cause for which they are retained. Although the parties may pay for the professional witness to prepare a report and to attend court, the witness is not a 'hired mouth' and must not be drawn into acting as an advocate for the cause of the client who pays him. Retain your impartiality and objectivity at all times. Remember that you owe an over-riding duty to the court.

### ▶ Never lose your temper

It is not difficult to feel irritated by proceedings in court. The delays, the stress, and other factors may make counsel's questions seem foolish or insulting. Remember that the trial is not necessarily a search for the truth, especially in civil cases. Both parties will be trying to win the case and although the counsel who calls you to give evidence will not usually try to undermine your evidence deliberately, the opponent's counsel will certainly be trying to do so if the evidence given is unfavourable to his client's case. By searching cross-examination, he will try to get you to concede points favourable to his case and to get you to agree with the position likely to be taken by the experts he calls.

However irritated you might feel, and however much you would like to finish and return to what you regard as a better use of your time, try never to let your irritation show, and never, ever, lose your temper. A 'rattled' witness is a gift to counsel and an intemperate expert witness is a positive danger to the judicial process. If the line of questioning really is unacceptable, the trial judge (or opposing counsel) is likely to intervene. Try to be calm and patient and to appear thoroughly professional, assisting the court to deal justly with the issues before it.

## References

1. Kapfunde *v* Abbey National PLC & Another [1998] CA Times Law Rep, 6 April
2. General Medical Council. *Confidentiality: Protecting and Providing Information.* London, 2000
3. W *v* Egdell [1990] 1 All ER 835
4. Arthur JS Hall & Co. *v* Simons [2000] 3 WLR 543
5. The Civil Procedure Rules. London: HMSO, 1998. www.open.gov.uk/lcd
6. *Access to Justice*. Final report of the Right Honourable Lord Woolf MR. London: HMSO, 1996
7. Cornelius *v* de Taranto [High Court decision; case No. 98-C-38; Nottingham Crown Court, 30 June 2000; Morland J.]
8. Expert Witness Institute, Africa House, Kingsway, London WC2B 6BG. Tel: 020 7745 7290; e-mail: info@EWI.org; URL: http://www.EWI.org.uk
9. Royal Society of Medicine. http://www.roysocmed.ad.uk
10. Medico-Legal Society. http://www.medico-legalsociety.org.uk

# ▶2

# The Doctor as Defendant

For many years, it has – sadly – been the case that few doctors can move from qualification to retirement without finding themselves defendants in legal proceedings of one kind or another. More and more statute law (ie laws passed by Parliament) is enacted which impinges on medical practice. There are 'over 500 references in UK statutes to the functions that may be performed by registered medical practitioners'.[1]

Doctors must obey all UK laws as much as any other citizen. Regulatory authorities are empowered to prosecute doctors for breaches of the law. Patients' organizations are ever more prepared to challenge doctors for their actions and for alleged transgressions of the law and codes of practice in a variety of fora, including the criminal courts and the GMC. Complaints against doctors are on the increase. For example, complaints to the GMC doubled in number from 1500 in 1995 to 3001 in 1999, and the GMC has a backlog of cases, despite its Professional Conduct Committee sitting for 129 days in 1999.[2]

I offer two pieces of advice to doctors. First, be sure to maintain membership of a medical protection and defence organization, for you will assuredly need help at some stage, and specialist advice and legal representation is seriously damaging to both health and wealth if it has to be funded from your usual income. Secondly, be sure to contact your medical protection and defence organization promptly and at an early opportunity if you face any kind of medico-legal challenge. Say nothing to anybody and do nothing until, first, you have taken some advice. Unwise statements made by doctors at an initial interview (at a time when they thought it was a simple matter and that there was nothing to worry about), before advice was taken, may be damning to a successful defence.

Doctors who face investigation by a statutory body including the police, their NHS Trust or Health Authority or other regulatory bodies are sometimes prone to open their mouths and to give statements *before* advice is taken. Some, not realizing that their conduct may be in breach of the law will thereby prejudice the prospects for a successful defence. It is better to make no comment and to give no statement until expert advice is taken, if there is any possibility that a prosecution or a disciplinary hearing might take place. Sound medico-legal advice and, where necessary and appropriate, legal representation can be provided, which protects the doctor's best interests.

English law is based on a presumption of innocence unless and until guilt is proven, beyond reasonable doubt, to the satisfaction of the court. There is no duty on the accused person to present the prosecutor with the evidence he needs to secure a conviction. It is for the prosecution to prove the guilt of the accused to the satisfaction of the court. So, do not condemn yourself from your own mouth. There is a right to remain silent in the face of investigation by the police and others – albeit that in certain circumstances adverse inferences may be drawn if an accused person does not say something in his defence at an appropriate stage. Your legal advisers will be able to advise you what to say and when and how to say it.

To recapitulate, seek expert medico-legal advice at the earliest opportunity whenever you face an inquiry that suggests that criminal or disciplinary proceedings against you are a real possibility. There is legal authority, in connection with the payment of taxes, that one is entitled to arrange one's financial affairs so as to *avoid* paying more tax than is legally required – but one may not *evade* paying taxes due because that is a criminal offence. So, in the context of professional medical conduct there is no legal duty on any doctor to assist the authorities by providing information that may help them to secure a conviction. One may remain silent, but it would be most unwise deliberately to mislead and it is, of course, a serious criminal offence to lie under oath. *Do* be frank and truthful with your own professional legal advisers, and then be guided by them as to how to respond to investigations and inquiries into your conduct.

## Crime and the defendant doctor: offences that may lead to prosecution

The common criminal offences for which a small number of doctors will, each year, face inquiries and criminal prosecutions include:

- Murder – usually in the context of 'euthanasia' or 'mercy killing'

- Manslaughter – usually in the context of gross negligence resulting in the death of a patient

- Indecent assault – ranging from inappropriate physical contact to rape

- Illegal abortion – rare in the UK since the implementation of the Abortion Act 1967

- ▶ Fraud and dishonesty – expenses claims, false prescriptions, etc.

- ▶ Perjury

- ▶ Fraud in research or clinical trials – with or without financial implications

- ▶ Misuse of drugs offences

- ▶ Genital mutilation – Prohibition of Female Circumcision Act 1985.

Regrettably, in the past half-century or so the teaching of legal principles and of forensic or legal medicine to medical undergraduate students has declined; and this at a time when more and more laws are passed which affect medical practice. Thus, many contemporary clinicians have an inadequate knowledge and understanding of the laws that govern their practices. It is to be hoped that those responsible for medical undergraduate and postgraduate education in the UK will come to appreciate not only the desirability but also the positive need for the return to the medical curriculum of some formal teaching of the law as it affects doctors.

A successful criminal prosecution requires two criteria: the prosecution must prove that the alleged unlawful act occurred (the *actus reus*); and that the act was accompanied by the necessary intent (the *mens rea*, or 'guilty mind', as it is sometimes known colloquially). Intent may be inferred from the nature of the act and surrounding circumstances. For example, you might find it difficult to persuade a jury that an intravenous bolus injection of potassium chloride alone was intended solely to relieve the pain of terminal carcinomatosis, even if you assert that that was your intention.

## 'A clean breast' – 'better to get it over and done with'

When a person is under investigation for an alleged criminal offence, the police and some defence lawyers may press them to admit the offence and to 'make a clean breast of it' and 'get it over and done with'. The matter is said to be relatively minor and court procedures and publicity are unwelcome; a guilty plea will be reflected in the punishment imposed, which will be less than if the matter is contested and the individual is found guilty after a trial, especially if it is a first offence.

Such inducements to plead guilty may be subtle. However, doctors must be most careful. If they are convicted of a criminal offence, especially one involving dishonesty, however seemingly 'trivial', the case will be reported to the GMC and the doctor will face an inquiry by them. The GMC takes a serious view of dishonesty and indeed of other criminal convictions involving doctors. Suspension or erasure from the Medical Register is a distinctly possible outcome.

Therefore, if you do not believe that you are guilty of the offence for which you are under investigation or with which you have been charged, either because you did not do the act or because you did not have the requisite intent, you should maintain your innocence and you should not plead guilty. As always, take early advice about your legal position and be guided by your legal advisers.

This chapter is not a text dealing with the criminal law; rather, it is concerned only with *medical evidence*. For a more detailed consideration of the law on these matters, the reader should look to other texts and sources of information. However, a summary will follow of some of the more important considerations about medical evidence in the principal crimes for which doctors are vulnerable.

## Murder

It is very important to avoid confusing *motive* with *intention*. Many doctors who treat terminally ill patients and who wish to relieve their suffering will receive requests, from the patient or the patient's relatives, to terminate their suffering. The doctor's motives may be of the highest, but the English law of murder is concerned with *intent*, not motive. If by your actions (eg administration of an excessive dose of an opiate drug which is swiftly followed by the death of the patient) you can be shown to have intended the shortening of life rather than the relief of pain or suffering, you will be seriously at risk of prosecution for murder. Murder, if proven, still carries a mandatory sentence of life imprisonment; the judge has no discretion over sentencing.

## Manslaughter

The leading medical case involving manslaughter is *R v Adomako*,[3] which arose from the death of a patient following an anaesthetic for an ophthalmic procedure. The issue in the appeal concerned the correct legal test for a jury to convict of manslaughter – was it to be the gross negligence test or the recklessness test? There was no question that the standard of care was below that which was to be expected – and thus ordinary civil negligence had occurred. However, were the anaesthetist's acts and omissions so reprehensible as to amount to a crime?

Despite the arguments put forward on behalf of Dr Adomako – that the law should be clear, certain, intellectually coherent and generally applicable and acceptable – the Lord Chancellor ruled that 'it is a sufficient direction to the jury to adopt the gross negligence test… and it is not necessary to refer to the definition of recklessness…' Thus, if the death of a patient arises from a doctor's negligence and a jury is of the view that the nature of the negligence was 'gross', a conviction for involuntary manslaughter might follow. No assistance has been offered by the House of Lords on how 'gross' is to be defined, except that it means 'really serious'. It is a matter for the jury to decide; they must consider whether any particular breach of duty should be characterized as gross negligence and therefore as a crime. The Lord Chancellor conceded that this 'to a certain extent involves an element of circularity' and observed that 'the essence of the matter... is whether having regard to the risk of death involved, the conduct of the defendant was so bad in all the circumstances as to amount in their judgement to a criminal act or omission'.

However, it may well be argued that this is less than helpful and that there is a real risk that a jury will confuse the seriousness of the act or omission with the seriousness of the consequences of the act or omission, especially in complex medical cases. Most clinicians will readily understand that many errors of a serious kind have relatively unimportant consequences and that some seemingly minor errors have the most profound consequences. If some assessment of recklessness is not to be part of the test for the jury, many other doctors will be seriously at risk of a conviction for manslaughter following a negligent error of the kind that would normally attract only civil compensation.

Any doctor who has the misfortune to be closely involved with the death of a patient following a negligent error is well advised to seek advice from his/her medical protection and defence organization at an early opportunity and before any statement is made to anyone other than their own medico-legal adviser. Whether or not a criminal investigation is undertaken and, if so, a criminal prosecution is brought against a practitioner will depend on many factors. Among the more important are, first, what the doctor says when questioned (hence the need to seek early advice, for many condemn themselves by their own premature and unwise utterances) and, secondly, what the experts consulted by the prosecuting authorities have to say (and hence the need for experts to act with care, skill and integrity). Generally, it is better not to fall down a hole than try to dig your way out of one, especially one dug by yourself. And if you do have the misfortune to find yourself in a hole, it is wise to stop digging at once. Instead, seek urgent advice.

## Indecent assault

Any unlawful touching of a person is an assault. If the touching is coupled with an act of indecency, a charge of indecent assault may follow. Doctors are especially vulnerable to complaints of alleged indecent assault and each year a small number of them face investigation. Many cases arise from misunderstanding; a few, sadly, from malicious complaints.

The alleged indecency may range from mere touching (eg hands allegedly brushing against the patient's breasts or thighs), through kissing to more serious matters such as clitoral stimulation during pelvic examinations, penile stimulation during genital examinations and unlawful sexual intercourse (often, allegedly, under the guise of some medical pretext). It is not unusual for there to be considerable delays (weeks or even months) between the alleged act and the visit from the police or other official representative. The doctor may have long forgotten the consultation and may be unable to recall the patient or the nature of the consultation. Good contemporaneous notes may be invaluable in preparing the doctor's defence; the absence of notes may make it very much more difficult to refute the allegations.

Doctors are usually devastated by an accusation of assault. In their anxiety to clear up the matter and to clear their name, they may start to speculate about what happened, or what 'must have happened'. The police may give a caution but the doctor, in his/her anxiety and believing his/her innocence, will speak at length, despite the caution and before seeking advice. It is not uncommon for doctors to make statements which they believe to be innocent or positively helpful in exonerating them but which in fact provide some corroborative evidence to the prosecuting authorities, enabling them to proceed to a criminal charge and prosecution.

Doctors who face this harrowing and unwelcome experience should lose no time in making prompt contact with their medico-legal advisers and should heed their advice.

Misunderstandings may arise when the patient is not expecting the doctor's actions or has misinterpreted his motives. A careful explanation before eliciting informed agreement to the proposed procedure would obviate many of the complaints. Three common examples are described below.

1.  A teenage girl attends a locum general practitioner with a complaint of sore throat. Without explaining why, he asks her to undress and proceeds to examine her chest and breasts. The doctor has noticed, from the medical records, that the patient is on the oral contraceptive pill and, being thorough, has decided to assess the breasts for lumps; but he has not explained his thoughts nor has he sought the patient's agreement. The patient did not expect to have her breasts examined and misunderstands the doctor's actions. She makes a formal complaint to the police who, later, arrest the doctor.

2.  A middle-aged woman is assessed by a doctor for a compensation claim following an accident. She complains of back pains. The doctor asks her to undress and, without explanation, examines her breasts. He wished to exclude breast carcinoma with bony secondaries as a possible differential

cause of her back pain. She believes that she has been abused and makes a complaint to police. The doctor is arrested and charged.

3. ENT and eye examinations can be misinterpreted if, without adequate explanation and consent, the clinician suddenly darkens the room, moves close to the patient (perhaps his thighs brushing hers) and comes 'cheek to cheek' in order to examine the eyes or ears. The patient believes that she has been indecently assaulted and complains.

Many complaints (but certainly not all) can be avoided if an explanation is given of what the doctor proposes and if the patient's consent is sought. It also may be helpful to have a chaperone (or at least to offer one to the patient) for some clinical assessments. As always, if a complaint is made, lose no time in contacting your medical protection and defence organization.

Occasionally, a fabricated or malicious complaint is made to the police. There may be many reasons for this – psychiatric illness, an attempt at blackmail, an attempt to redress some perceived slight or grievance, an opportunistic attempt to gain press and media publicity and to sell a story for profit, to name but a few. The doctor's medical protection and defence organizations are well placed to help in all these situations and should be contacted promptly by any doctor facing a complaint.

Of course, some complaints of indecency are well-founded and may be upheld when the matter comes to trial. Such doctors bring shame on themselves, their family and the profession, and inevitably, after a conviction, face disciplinary proceedings before the Professional Conduct Committee of the GMC, which takes a serious view of breaches of trust between doctors and patients. Suspension or erasure from the Medical Register is a likely additional sanction for the errant doctor, over and above any sanction imposed by the Crown Court.

## Illegal abortion

It is now rare in Great Britain for a doctor to face a prosecution for illegal abortion, for there is no need to break the law since the enactment of the Abortion Act 1967. However, it is important to comply with the provisions of the Act (as amended) and Regulations, particularly concerning the statutory certification and reporting requirements.

## Fraud and dishonesty

Doctors are expected to act responsibly and to be trustworthy, for they have been granted many statutory and other privileges as registered medical practitioners. Their signatures on a variety of forms and certificates may lead to the expenditure of considerable sums of public money. They are expected to exercise appropriate care over everything to which they append their signatures and over statements that they make and upon which others will rely. Common sources of difficulty are sickness certificates (both statutory and private), prescriptions for medicines (especially for persons living abroad or wanting them to take abroad or for family members abroad) and passport applications. Care must also be taken in claiming expenses.

If a doctor is shown to have acted dishonestly or with intention to defraud or deceive, he/she may face criminal prosecution with a real risk, on conviction, not only of imprisonment or fine but also of further action by the GMC, which takes a very serious view of this kind of dishonesty. A criminal conviction may well lead to suspension or erasure from the Medical Register.

Paperwork may be a chore and innocent mistakes may arise, especially by doctors who accord it low priority. However, there is a professional obligation to act correctly, carefully and responsibly. If a doctor faces inquiry, advice should be taken at once. It might be relatively easy for a prosecutor to prove the *act* necessary for the crime (the doctor's signature on the piece of paper is there for all to see) but the doctor's *intention* may not be clear cut – and both elements are necessary in English law in order to secure a conviction. Thus, take advice before making any statement. Depending on the facts and circumstances of the particular case, it may be possible to argue that the doctor's intention was not to deceive. However, the law on dishonesty is complex and the court may be entitled to draw inferences about the intention of the accused from his/her actions; so, it might not be sufficient simply to argue, 'yes, it might be my signature but I did not mean it to deceive...'

## Perjury

It is a serious criminal offence to give false evidence under oath or affirmation. Tempting though it may be – and honourable though it might appear to some – to try to assist a colleague who is in difficulty by giving 'supportive' evidence, giving false evidence is wrong and may lead to a criminal charge under the Perjury Act 1911.

Prosecutions of doctors for perjury are rare but not unknown, usually when one doctor gives false evidence in a court (including a Coroner's Court) in a misguided effort to get a colleague 'off the hook' following the death of a patient, or in support of one or other party in a civil matter such as a compensation claim or a divorce or child custody case.

Experts, too, must take great care to ensure that their evidence – whether oral or written – is correct in all material particulars. In civil cases in England

and Wales, the Civil Procedure Rules (CPR) make it clear that experts owe an over-riding duty to the *court*. They must not dissemble or deceive.

## Research

Fraud or dishonesty in research has been a source of grave concern in recent years. There may be a variety of pressures on researchers to publish original research, or to participate in post-marketing surveillance of medicines. Some doctors have yielded to the temptation to falsify results, whether for financial advantage or other reasons. Such conduct is ethically reprehensible and may well lead to a criminal prosecution. It will also result in an investigation by the GMC.

## Misuse of drugs

Quite apart from any temptation by doctors to misuse controlled drugs personally or 'recreationally', they face prosecution under the Misuse of Drugs legislation if their prescribing is other than properly *bona fide* or if they do not keep their supplies of drugs securely or their drugs registers up to date. Some doctors have yielded to the temptation to supply controlled drugs to 'patients' in return for money or for sexual favours. Such conduct will lead not only to prosecution but also to subsequent inquiry by the GMC.

It is important to comply strictly with the provisions of the law concerning the supply and safe-keeping of controlled drugs. It will be easier to prepare a defence to alleged offences if doctors keep good evidence in the form of contemporaneous notes and records and maintain their drug register properly.

## Genital mutilation

Following an outcry some years ago about genital surgical procedures on young women and girls, some (but by no means all) of which were undertaken by medically registered practitioners, the Prohibition of Female Circumcision Act 1985 was enacted. This places very strict controls on genital procedures and the circumstances under which and by whom they may be performed. Non-compliance with the provisions of the Act may lead to criminal prosecution but there is unlikely to be a problem for medical practitioners who provide demonstrably necessary treatments for pathological conditions.

## Miscellaneous

There are many other ways in which doctors may find themselves having to give evidence in connection with their defence in criminal matters and breaches of statutory regulations. In some cases, the alleged offences will arise from the practice of the doctors' profession and they may then approach their medical protection and defence organizations for help. In other cases, the alleged offences will arise not from their professional practice but simply as citizens, and in those cases they should consult their personal solicitors, legal expenses insurer or motoring organization, etc.

In general and in conclusion, doctors who face criminal charges or serious disciplinary proceedings should:

▶ remain silent until appropriate advice is obtained

▶ contact their medical protection and defence organizations or other appropriate legal advisers as soon as possible

▶ make a detailed, written record of all relevant facts as soon as possible, retaining it for the use of their own legal adviser so that the statement remains legally privileged

## The doctor as defendant in civil proceedings

For most doctors, the threat of civil proceedings, usually for alleged medical negligence, is much more common than implication in criminal proceedings. However, a claim for compensation can be seriously damaging to both health and wealth. The wise and prudent doctor will take care to maintain appropriate membership of a medical protection and defence organization.

This is important even for doctors who are employed by NHS Trusts and Health Authorities. Although the indemnity scheme known as 'Crown indemnity' operates for employed NHS staff[4] (but not for independent contractors such as GPs), it only provides cover for the management and financing of medical negligence claims arising strictly from the performance of the employee's duties under his or her contract with the NHS. The 'Crown indemnity' scheme does not cover employees for private work of any kind, nor for 'good samaritan' acts, disciplinary matters, defamation, GMC hearings, etc. Your employer will not necessarily be concerned to uphold your professional reputation, nor be willing to resolve disputes such as those between different employees.

Doctors in independent practice (including NHS general practice where they are contracted to provide services but are not 'employees') are required to make their own indemnity arrangements. That is now a professional obligation under the GMC Rules.[5] The Health Act 1999 also contains a statutory provision for the Secretary of State to make regulations requiring clinicians to have professional indemnity insurance but (at the time of writing) no such regulations had been made.

## Early intimations

You may realize that litigation against you is 'on the cards' in a variety of ways. First, you may recognize that you have perpetrated some error and, if you do, you should report the matter promptly to your medical protection or defence organization, or to your manager in your NHS Trust or Health Authority. Second, you may receive a request for disclosure of the patient's medical records. Third, you may receive correspondence direct from the patient, the patient's relatives or the patient's legal advisers requesting information. Finally, it is now increasingly common for treating clinicians to know about a medical accident before the patient does, because of the introduction of risk management adverse incident reporting systems. However you are alerted to the potential for civil litigation, you should lose no time in reporting the matter promptly to your defence body and (if you are an NHS employee) to your employer's claims manager or legal department.

Patients and those who advise them have a statutory entitlement to relevant health records.[6] The usual procedure in England and Wales will be for the patient's advisers to obtain copies of the clinical records and to take expert advice from medical experts and legal counsel. If the facts are believed to give rise to a sustainable claim, legal proceedings are likely to be commenced.

If the treatment was provided in the hospital or community health sectors of the NHS, the likelihood is that the claimant will sue the NHS Trust as defendant and the individual practitioner may not be named as a defendant; but if the treatment was provided by a 'private', independent clinician, the clinician may well be named as defendant. It is important, then, for the defendant(s) to act promptly, putting the matter in the hands of their legal adviser or medical protection and defence organizations so that a defence is formulated. Failure to act promptly may mean that judgment is entered against the defendant in default.

In the space available, it is not possible to deal with the detail of the civil justice litigation process; but the 'take-home message' is that such litigation must not be 'treated conservatively' (ie ignored) in the hope that it will be self-limiting (ie 'go away'). It must be regarded as malign and treated with urgency and with determination by the claims experts (the doctor's or Trust's legal advisers).

## Prompt reporting

You are advised to make a full, written report at the earliest opportunity, documenting the full facts in chronological order. Litigation, even since the reforms to civil justice made in the wake of the Woolf Report,[7] is a slow process; it may be months or years before the case is adjudicated. Facts fade from the memory, or are subject to imperfect recall, all too swiftly. Better to make a full, contemporaneous note whilst the events are fresh in the memory.

## Defence of a claim

The defence team will review the clinical records, the various statements and will seek expert opinion upon the defensibility or otherwise of the claim. If the claim is believed to be indefensible, a settlement will usually be negotiated – but if it is not possible to agree mutually acceptable terms for a settlement, the case may go to court. Sometimes liability may be disputed, sometimes liability may be conceded but the harm alleged to have arisen as a direct consequence of the alleged negligence is in dispute. Sometimes both liability and the amount of harm or damages payable may be disputed. If the case cannot be settled 'out of court', there might be lengthy delays before it comes to court, even since the reforms to civil justice and the CPR.[8] The preparation of a successful defence is detailed and time-consuming; it requires the sympathetic cooperation of all those who played a part in the clinical care.

Owing to limitations on space in this book, the reader is referred to other sources of information about the handling of clinical negligence claims, such as from his or her medical protection and defence organization, NHS Trust legal department, medical association or the literature (eg articles in the literature, including the journal *Clinical Risk\**).

## Other torts

A tort is a civil wrong. For the doctor, the most common example is medical negligence, but s/he might become embroiled in other civil claims such as defamation – libel and slander. An accurate report in a journal, newspaper or broadcast medium will probably not be actionable. However, inaccurate reports or any statements which tend to lower the esteem of another person in the minds of 'right-thinking' people might give rise to an actionable claim. Responsible professional criticism may be defensible but inaccurate comments or irresponsible, pejorative remarks about others might leave the speaker or writer open to an action for defamation.

At least one of the UK defence bodies has stated that it will not usually assist members with defamation proceedings and all the defence bodies are very circumspect about providing assistance in connection with litigation for libel and slander. So, take great care over what you state or write, and if you write for a

*RSM Press, 1 Wimpole Street, London W1G 0AE; 020 7290 3916.

living (medical journalism, etc.) be sure to take out adequate insurance for defamation actions. Space here does not permit an account of the relevant law. Doctors who need to learn more should consult other texts. Anyone facing a claim as a defendant in civil proceedings should take expert legal advice at the earliest opportunity – 'a doctor who attempts to manage his own claim has a fool for a client and an incompetent for a lawyer,' it is said, and with good reason.

## The doctor as defendant in disciplinary proceedings

As well as the criminal and civil courts, doctors are professionally accountable to a variety of disciplinary and other professional bodies. These include the GMC, the employer (whether NHS Trust, NHS Health Authority and independent sector) and medical Royal Colleges. Independent contractors in the NHS (general practitioners) and elsewhere (eg those with admitting privileges in private clinics and hospitals but who are not employees) will also have to be prepared to answer to a variety of accountability procedures.

Perhaps the most feared tribunal is the GMC, since that has the power to remove a practitioner's registration and, therefore, his/her ability to earn a living as a registered medical practitioner. The GMC itself now has more than one tribunal to which a doctor may be accountable. The Health Committee and the Professional Conduct Committee procedures have been joined by a procedure to review a chronic pattern of poor performance, and currently there is a proposal to add a requirement for periodic reaccreditation.

Space in this book precludes a consideration of each procedure. A doctor faced with a complaint about his or her professional work, or one accused of any sort of professional impropriety, and called to account for his/her actions should treat the matter with seriousness and urgency. What might seem to the individual clinician to be absurd, preposterous or inconsequential may turn out to have the most profound consequences for his/her registration or future employment prospects. The only safe and sensible course is to seek, urgently, advice from those best placed to provide it, such as a medical protection and defence organization, a medical association or a specialist lawyer with experience in medico-legal cases.

## References

1. General Medical Council. *Revalidating Doctors: Ensuring Standards, Securing the Future* [Summary]. London, July 2000: 10, para 36
2. General Medical Council. *GMC News* July 2000; issue 1

3.   R *v* Adomako [1995] 1 AC 171; House of Lords, 30 June 1994
4.   NHS Department of Health. Circular HC(89)34
5.   GMC. *Good Medical Practice*, paragraph 20. London, July 1998
6.   Access to Health Records Act 1990
7.   *Access to Justice: Final Report*. The Rt. Hon. Lord Woolf MR. London: The Stationery Office, 1996. ISBN 0-11-3800991
8.   Civil Procedure Rules. London: The Stationery Office. URL www.open.gov.uk/lcd

# ▶3
# Evidence in the Coroner's Court

Coroners in England and Wales are independent judicial officers who hold office under the Crown and who are solely responsible, subject to the requirements of the law, for the conduct of their duties. A different system operates in Scotland. The law governing Coroners is set out in the Coroners Act 1988, the Treasure Act 1996 and in the Coroners Rules 1984 and other statutory instruments.

Coroners must be qualified legally or medically and of at least five-year's standing in their profession. There are some 148 Coroner's districts; and most Coroners are part-time and are solicitors. Some are barristers and a few are medical practitioners. There are about 26 full-time Coroners, in the big cities. Only a very few Coroners are qualified in law as well as medicine. Each Coroner must appoint a deputy Coroner and may appoint also an assistant deputy Coroner.

A Coroner may be under a duty to hold an inquest if there is a body lying within his district and the death has been violent or unnatural, sudden with an unknown cause, or has occurred in prison or in a place or in circumstances such as to require an inquest. In certain specified circumstances, a Coroner must hold the inquest before a jury (of between seven and 11 persons, not 12 as with criminal jury trials).

Coroners' courts in England and Wales are different from all other English courts because their proceedings are inquisitorial. Other courts, both criminal and civil, are accusatorial and adversarial – there are parties or 'sides' who are represented by counsel, and one or other party is trying to 'win' by persuading a judge or jury to find in their favour.

In Coroners' courts, there are no 'sides' and no 'parties', and no one is on trial. The usual protections for witnesses and the usual rules of evidence in civil and criminal courts do not apply in the same way. The Coroner conducts an inquiry, known as an inquisition, on behalf of Her Majesty the Queen. A Coroner's function and powers are strictly limited by statute.[1] When a Coroner is informed that the body of a person is lying within his jurisdiction[2] and there is reasonable cause to suspect that the deceased died an unnatural death, a sudden death of which the cause is unknown or has died in certain places (such as a prison or whilst in police custody), he/she must hold an inquest into the death of the deceased.[3]

All inquests must be held in public.[4] The sole purpose of an inquest is to establish and to record in the inquisition, which must be in writing and under the hand of the Coroner, who the deceased was and how, when and where the deceased came by his/her death.[5] 'How' simply means 'by what means'; it does not mean a detailed inquiry into the background and surrounding circumstances.

If a deceased person was attended by his doctor in his last illness and the doctor is able to issue a medical certificate of the cause of death that is accepted by the Registrar of Deaths, the Coroner has no interest or jurisdiction. But if the death is violent or unnatural or sudden with cause unknown, the death will be reported to the Coroner. Usually, a Coroner's postmortem examination is arranged, performed by a pathologist, to try to establish a medical cause of death. If the death appears to have been the result of a crime, a forensic pathologist approved for the purpose (a 'Home Office pathologist') will conduct a 'special' postmortem examination.

Often, a Coroner will be able to conclude matters following a postmortem examination that establishes that the medical cause of death was 'natural', by issuing the appropriate certificate to enable the Registrar of Deaths to register the death. However, if this is not possible, an inquest will be arranged and evidence will be presented, some of it written and some of it – usually, but not invariably – oral.

Some deaths must, by statute, be the subject of an inquest with a jury,[6] such as deaths in prison or in police custody. Curiously, there is no statutory obligation to summon a jury for the death in hospital of a patient detained compulsorily under an Order of the Mental Health Act 1983; however, there is a non-statutory Home Office 'recommendation' that such deaths might be the subject of an inquest with a jury.[7]

Coroners no longer have, as they once did, a power to make a finding of unlawful killing (murder, manslaughter or infanticide) against a named individual, committing him for trial on the verdict of the Coroner. The last such case in England and Wales involving a medical practitioner was that of *R v Rai* in Cardiff in 1978. (In this case, the junior doctor was acquitted, but not before the emotional trauma of a full jury trial in the Crown Court.) Now, statute[8] provides that the proceedings and evidence at an inquest shall be directed solely to ascertaining who the deceased was and how, when and where the deceased came by his death; and neither the Coroner nor the jury shall express any opinion on any other matter. No verdict may be framed in such a way as to appear to determine any question of criminal liability on the part of a named person or civil liability.[9]

A Coroner may, at the conclusion of an inquest and in appropriate cases, return a verdict of 'unlawful killing' without naming any person. If he believes that action should be taken to prevent the recurrence of fatalities similar to that in respect of which the inquest was held, the Coroner may report the matter in writing to the person or authority who may have power to take such action.[10]

## Evidence for the inquest

The detailed practice varies from Coroner to Coroner. Most will conduct their preliminary inquiries through Coroners' officers, who are often serving police officers but may come from a wide range of backgrounds. They will receive the initial notification to the Coroner, often from a medical practitioner. Doctors who were involved in the care of a person in a case reported to the Coroner may be asked to submit a statement.

If the doctor's statement is detailed and accurate and contains the relevant facts that the Coroner needs to decide 'who, how, when and where', it might not be necessary to call the doctor to the Coroner's court to give oral evidence. It may be possible for the Coroner to read the statement in court. However, if the statement is incomplete, or omits key dates and facts, the Coroner will have no alternative but to call the doctor to give oral evidence. It also may be necessary for the Coroner to call the doctor if interested persons,[11] such as a parent, spouse or personal representative of the deceased or a beneficiary under a policy of insurance, an insurer, etc., wish to examine a witness.

Reports to Coroners should be written in the active voice, making clear the role of the author of the report (his qualifications, position held, his part in the care of the patient, and so on) and should set out the facts clearly, logically and chronologically. Make clear the difference between what *you* did and what was done by others. Coroners, usually through their officers, will gather statements from all persons who had a part to play and whose evidence may be relevant to the purpose of the inquest. A date will then be set for the inquest, and the Coroner will decide which witnesses to call.

## At the inquest

If you are called to give evidence, in most cases you are unlikely to require legal representation; but you may always seek advice from your medical protection or defence organization. A decision to hold an inquest does not imply, of itself, that anyone's conduct will be criticized – and of course no verdict may appear to determine criminal liability on the part of a named person or civil liability.

If, during the proceedings, an interested person attempts to ask questions of a witness which are not relevant or which attempt to impute liability, the Coroner will intervene to prevent the question being pursued. No witness at an inquest is required to answer any question tending to incriminate him/herself.[12] Where any person's conduct is called into question at an inquest on grounds which the Coroner thinks substantial and which relate to the purpose of the inquest (to establish who, when, where and how the deceased came by his death), and that person is not present, the Coroner has the power to adjourn the inquest so that the individual may be present.[13]

Unnecessary legal representation of a witness at an inquest, especially a medical witness, may be counterproductive in that it arouses suspicion in the minds of the Coroner and of others that the witness has something to fear or hide, which is seldom the case. It is worth re-stating here that an inquest is *not* a trial; it is an inquisitorial process to establish the identity of the deceased and how, where and when he/she came by his/her death. 'How', the court has ruled,[14] simply means 'by what means'. It is not a wide-ranging public inquiry into all the background circumstances.

Increasingly, various pressure groups and others attempt to use inquest proceedings for other purposes; sometimes to pursue a campaign of one kind or another. Coroners increasingly are subjected to challenges by way of Judicial Review applications in respect of the decisions that they reach. In this, they share the burden of many professional people in increasingly litigious times. However, the purpose of an inquest is simple enough and doctors should seldom have problems in their dealings with Coroners if the basic rules of evidence are followed and the purpose of an inquest is borne in mind.

## The 'verdict'

Coroners, having conducted an inquest, with or without a jury, will return a 'verdict'. The 'verdict' is, in fact, the whole of the formal inquisition findings, which includes the name, date of birth, address, occupation and medical cause of death of the deceased, as well as what is commonly thought of as the 'verdict'; that is, the conclusion – that death was natural or was the result of unlawful killing, accident, suicide, industrial disease, abuse of drugs, etc.

Verdicts of unlawful killing (ie murder, manslaughter or infanticide) may be returned if the evidence warrants it and meets the stricter, criminal standard of proof – 'satisfied so that you are sure' or 'beyond reasonable doubt'. The same strict test applies to conclusions that the deceased killed himself – the intention to do so has to be present at the time the act is done. All other conclusions are reached on the less strict standard of proof applicable in civil cases – that is, on 'the balance of probability'. Where the Coroner (or jury) cannot be sure of the conclusion, an 'open' verdict should be returned.

Doctors should note that unlawful killing includes 'gross negligence manslaughter'. They should also note that, in appropriate cases and where the evidence supports it, a Coroner or Coroner's jury may include 'neglect' as part of the verdict and this is sometimes relevant in medical cases. In this context, readers are referred also to comments in the previous two chapters.

## Statistics

Every Coroner is required by law to make annual returns in writing to the Secretary of State (Home Office), providing 'such particulars as the Secretary of State may direct' about the cases in which they have held an inquest. The data are published by the Home Office from time to time.

In 1997, 190 000 deaths in England and Wales were reported to Coroners – some 34% of all deaths that year. Of those, 88% were concluded without inquest and only 12% of the deaths reported to Coroners resulted in an inquest. Nearly half of those resulted in a verdict of accidental death; other common verdicts were suicide, natural causes, industrial disease and 'open'.

## Scotland

The law in Scotland is different from that in other parts of the UK. There are no Coroners and no inquests in Scotland. Instead, deaths that would be reportable to Coroners in other parts of the UK are dealt with by the Procurators Fiscal and by the Sheriffs, and what would be called an inquest in other parts of the UK is known as a 'Fatal Accident Inquiry' in Scotland. Insofar as medical evidence is concerned, however, the underlying principles set out above are not dissimilar.

## References

1. Coroners Act 1988; The Coroners Rules, 1984 (SI [1984]) No. 552 (as amended)
2. Coroners Act 1988, section 5(1)
3. Coroners Act 1988, section 8(1)
4. The Coroners Rules 1984, rule 17
5. Coroners Act 1988, section 11(5)
6. Coroners Act 1988, section 8(3)

7. Home Office Circular, No. 35, 1969
8. The Coroners Rules 1984, rule 36
9. The Coroners Rules 1984, rule 42
10. The Coroners Rules 1984, rule 43
11. The Coroners Rules 1984, rule 20 (as amended)
12. The Coroners Rules 1984, 22
13. The Coroners Rules 1984, 24
14. R *v* HM Coroner for North Humberside & Scunthorpe ex p. Jamieson [1995] 1 QB 1

# ►4
# Doctors and Tribunals

## Introduction

Doctors may, from time to time, be called upon to appear before tribunals as medical witnesses. Although less formal than courts of law, giving professional evidence in tribunals, either of fact or expert opinion, is often crucial to the issues under consideration. These tribunals exercise their jurisdiction with wide discretion, applying the principles of natural justice in a manner unfettered by the strict application of rules of law.

For the purposes of this chapter, I shall use the employment tribunal as a model. There are, however, some eighty jurisdictions, the majority of which will not require medical evidence and others may only require production of documentary evidence.

In this chapter, I will briefly review the use of tribunals in general and the employment tribunal in particular. Later, I will concentrate on the giving of evidence.

## General aspects of tribunals

In its most general sense, a 'tribunal' is any person or body of persons empowered to judge or adjudicate, or determine claims and disputes. Today, the term is applied to a person or body of persons who form what was formerly known as 'administrative tribunals'. These are quite distinct from courts, where professional judges preside, and formal procedures and decisions are made according to the strict rules of law.

The number, variety and jurisdictions of tribunals has expanded considerably since the end of the First World War, such that questions are now being asked – mainly by academic lawyers – as to whether the present trend can be allowed to continue. Tribunals were originally established to:

▶ decide issues not wholly suitable to courts of law

▶ bring experience and subject expertise to the decision, and

▶ operate locally, speedily and cheaply.

The principal reasons that this trend should be allowed to continue, therefore, are to increase access to the law and to ensure that the decisions made within these tribunals are appropriate to modern society.

Tribunals have certain common features, which include:

▶ a composition, largely or entirely, of lay persons

▶ often a legally qualified Chair

▶ simplicity and informality of procedure, and

▶ decisions based on discretion, impression and experience, rather than the rules of law.

Appeals to a court are restricted or practically excluded. Where they *are* allowed, they are usually confined to questions of law. Most tribunals are subject to the supervision of the Council on Tribunals insofar as non-judicial matters are concerned (eg policy, training, etc.), and to the supervisory jurisdiction of the courts. This ensures that the tribunal observes the rules of natural justice and does not act *ultra vires* or otherwise unlawfully.

## Tribunals and the law of employment

Several situations might require the appearance of a doctor before an employment tribunal. The doctor may be a respondent to a claim against him/herself from one of his/her staff, or, more likely, he/she may be called upon as a witness, either to fact or as an expert.

Employment rights are regulated partly by the law of contract and partly by statute, of which the most important is the Employment Rights Act 1996. Tribunals also have jurisdiction under other, often anti-discrimination, legislation, including:

▶ The Equal Pay Act 1970

▶ The Sex Discrimination Acts 1975 and 1986

▶ The Race Relations Act 1976, and

▶ The Disability Discrimination Act 1995.

Actions for breach of contract are usually pursued in the High Court or County Court, where legal representation and legal aid is available. Statutes confer jurisdiction on the employment tribunals for all other matters concerned with unfair dismissal and anti-discrimination laws. These tribunals comprise a legally qualified Chair and two laypersons representing employers and trade unions. The process is relatively informal, and legal aid is not available to an applicant. However, legal representation is unnecessary and the parties are represented frequently by trade union officials and human resource managers, depending on the complexity of the case. Each party bears their own costs unless the tribunal considers that the case has been brought or defended unreasonably.

Appeal lies on a point of law to the Employment Appeals Tribunal (EAT), which is composed of a High Court judge and two laypersons, as in the 'inferior' tribunals. The EAT sits in London and Glasgow; legal aid is available and further appeals lie to the Court of Appeal and the House of Lords.

When an application is made before a tribunal, the Advisory, Conciliation and Arbitration Service (ACAS) will offer its services to the parties. Most applications are dropped as a result of the effectiveness of this procedure. Their 'award' is not usually legally binding.

The Industrial Relations Act 1971 introduced the concept of unfair dismissal and has had significant effects on employee relations generally. The principles of natural justice must be applied. An employer dismissing an employee must give a reason and be prepared to defend it at tribunal. The employee must be warned, allowed to put their side of the story and be given an opportunity to improve before action is taken against them. These, then, are the principles of unfair dismissal.

An employee may be dismissed in any one of three ways. He may be told to go with or without notice; he may be informed that the fixed-term contract on which he is employed will not be renewed when it expires, or he may be the subject of constructive dismissal. The employer dismisses constructively when he behaves in a way that constitutes such a breach of his side of the contract of employment that the employee is justified in terminating the relationship. An employer constructively dismisses an employee when he puts the employee's health or safety at risk so that the employee resigns.

Occasionally, a constructive dismissal, like dismissal with notice or summary dismissal, is not necessarily unfair. A supervisor of a packing department, who had been off sick, was told that he would have to move to the job of production foreman. He refused on the grounds that it would damage his health and would not agree to a medical examination to assess his suitability. He resigned. He had been constructively dismissed because the employer had no contractual right to move him to another job, without his consent. But the employer acted reasonably and was not liable for unfair dismissal.

The employee has to prove that he has been dismissed. If he does so, the burden shifts to the employer to give a reason; the tribunal then decides whether, in all the circumstances, he acted reasonably in dismissing the individual. They will need to be convinced that the employer acted within a range of reasonable responses. They do not need to be persuaded that, given the circumstances, they would have reached the same conclusion.

The Employment Rights Act 1996 lists five possible groups of fair reasons:

- Capability or qualifications, capability being assessed by reference to skill, aptitude, health or any other physical or mental quality

- Misconduct

- Redundancy (that is, that the employee's job will disappear)

- That the employee cannot continue in employment without contravention of a statute

- Some other substantial reason.

In addition, the tribunal has to ask whether, based on the facts, the employer acted justly. For a decision to dismiss for dishonesty to be considered fair, there must be some evidence to act as the basis for the employer's decision.

The Act provides that size and administrative resources of the employer's undertaking are to be taken into account in deciding what is reasonable. Doctors are most likely to be involved with these tribunals under the heading of 'capability', possibly 'contravention of a statute' or 'some other substantial reason'.

Dismissal on the grounds of ill health is a very difficult area indeed, because the employee may well lose his/her job for something that is clearly not his/her fault. The leading case on dismissal for ill health is *East Lindsey District Council v Daubney*).[1] In this case, a surveyor employed by the Council was dismissed following prolonged periods of absence due to anxiety and general debility. Medical advice was sought from the District Community Physician, who wrote that the employee was unfit to carry out his duties and should be retired on the grounds of permanent ill health. The council acted on this information, without indicating to the employee that his job might be at risk or allowing him to obtain his own doctor's report. Dismissal was held to be unfair.

Generally, it is expected that employers obtain medical evidence before taking such decisions. This is both to assess the potential for return to work and the likely capability of the employee if he is allowed to return. It is also advisable for a manager to interview the employee in person, or at least communicate by post to ask how he feels about coming back and to warn him that the employer is considering dismissal.

Consulting the employee allows the true medical position to be ascertained, the employment situation to be assessed and a consideration of whether the employee could be offered ill-health retirement or a different job more suited to his condition. An employer is not obliged to artificially create work for a sick employee, however deserving his case.

Distinguishing between ill health and misconduct is the biggest single problem. To be absent from work through illness is not misconduct, but failure to turn up for work with no good reason is. Disciplinary procedures are inappropriate in genuine ill-health cases. But employees who have recurrent short-term absences, all ostensibly for medical reasons, usually trivial and unrelated ones, and never of sufficient duration to need medical certification, are usually managed with procedures similar to the disciplinary rules. With this background, it is now time to turn to the main thrust of this chapter, which covers the appearance before tribunals.

## The hearing

Much of the preparatory casework before an employment tribunal is carried out by individuals who are not necessarily legally qualified. They should, however, have been well trained in procedure. If further particulars, answers to questions or unearthing of documents are required, the parties or their representative may apply to an employment tribunal or seek a hearing for directions. A hearing for directions may:

- clarify the claims and issues

- make orders for unearthing and exchange of statements, and

- order a pre-hearing review or a preliminary hearing, and fix the date, time and place of that hearing.

Medical witnesses – and witnesses in general – are not really required at pre-hearing reviews. They are designed to determine if any matter being put forward has a reasonable prospect of success. If it has not, the pre-hearing review may order payment of a deposit from the applicant and give warnings about costs, etc. Preliminary hearings involve jurisdictional matters, such as whether the tribunal has jurisdiction in the applicant's claim. This may happen, for example, if the claim is out of time or if the claim is already litigated or settled. Witnesses at preliminary hearings are restricted to these points alone. Medical evidence is only rarely required.

The last type of hearing is a full-merits hearing, where the cases are prepared in advance. The course of such hearings is fairly standard. Initial matters are discussed, issues are identified, documents are produced and relevant law is identified. Presentation of the applicant's case, and cross-examination of the applicant's witnesses, follow. The respondent's witnesses then undergo examination (chief examination, cross-examination and re-examination), and the case closes with final submissions.

Cross-examination (ie questioning from the other side) is likely as in any court of law, to attempt to make the doctor appear unclear, inconsistent, misleading or irrelevant.

## Preparation

There are certain things that one should not do as a medical witness at a tribunal. Arriving late will no doubt lead to a rebuke from the Chair and do nothing to enhance one's professional image. The Chair will also be irritated if one frequently has to look up in one's notes to verify the simplest facts. Whether the applicant was on Voltarol or not is something which the physician or expert witness ought to know. This matters if you are giving expert evidence or, indeed, professional evidence of fact.

Displaying one's weaknesses simply offers an open door at cross-examination and might be seen as demonstrating a lack of competence.

It is not permissible for the medical witness to lose his/her temper as the questions become increasingly difficult during the tribunal, even if he/she has had a terrible time crossing the city to get to the tribunal venue. Losing one's temper is, in effect, playing into the examiner or cross-examiner's hands, as indeed will hasty answers made without thought or care. This will stoke what has been very aptly called the 'fires of discomfort'.

The secret of giving good evidence is in acquiring good basic techniques and in careful preparation.

▶ Know the details of the case thoroughly, as well as where in the file one might find appropriate references. There will be an agreed bundle and you should be familiar with its contents.

▶ Ensure that you have sufficient knowledge of the facts of the case, as well as any relevant literature. As far as employment tribunals are concerned, professional witnesses to fact will have a far easier time. Expert evidence, increasingly used today in applications under the Disability Discrimination Act 1995, will need to have a much wider knowledge of the relevant literature, similar in many ways to the practice in higher courts.

Experience, naturally, increases confidence. One's performance in the witness box will be open to comment by the tribunal, and such comments, particularly if adverse, are likely to find their way into the local or national press. However, giving evidence is a lot like sport. Prowess improves with practice. Obviously, experience will increase one's confidence.

## Going to the tribunal

Several week's notice of the tribunal date is usually given. Few take the opportunity to prepare, arriving at the tribunal readied for their duties. It is worthwhile to take some time and trouble over preparation at this stage, no matter how trivial the evidence appears to be. It is important that you check all the relevant notes, reports, documents, X-rays and any other material that relates to your evidence. Re-check the notes and reports. Although it is unnecessary to commit the reports to memory, as the Chair will allow reference to them whilst you are in the witness box, it is well to have the principal facts in mind. As you are being led through your statement, it is quite likely that you will misread a measurement or a similar fact. A polite and immediate correction will demonstrate that you are in control of the situation. It will also indicate that attempts to discredit one's knowledge of the facts are likely to be unsuccessful. In other words, it is a defensive sign against attack from those about to question you.

Finally, a reasonable knowledge of any medical conditions that have a bearing on the case is absolutely essential. An hour spent reading through the appropriate chapter in a relevant book will undoubtedly improve one's confidence, even if it is the night before.

There is much time spent waiting around in a tribunal room and it would almost be advisable for you to have a small book on any relevant subject in your briefcase. It is interesting how, before you go into the tribunal room, your mind concentrates on the issues at hand.

Because the matter is being handled by a tribunal and not by a court of law, the issues should not be regarded as trivial. Any experienced witness will be able to recall the way that they learnt this lesson in the past, often to their cost. The very fact that a doctor is being called to give either professional or expert evidence should always trigger a warning of storms ahead. Your presence there carries with it a price tag, and thus you are there for a good reason. Even if this reason is unknown, it is appropriate to have a few counter-measures at your disposal, such as the small but very relevant textbook in your briefcase or the latest review. The key to being a good tribunal witness therefore is *preparation, preparation, preparation*, to paraphrase one well-known barrister.

## Arriving at the tribunal

The quality of your evidence is likely to be unaffected by your faded jeans, open-necked shirt and the like; however, if you are badly dressed, you are less likely to be taken seriously by the members of the tribunal and hence your evidence will not be considered for what it is worth. Often, they will see it as a discourtesy to the tribunal for a professional person to attend in such casual attire. Your overall appearance will influence the opinion that the tribunal will have of your abilities and competence.

Given that the tribunal is usually chaired by an experienced lawyer and supported by two wing members from the Trade's Union Congress and the Confederation of British Industry, it can be suggested, with some considerable support, that the public still expect their professionals to look the part.

It has also been suggested that the professional who has taken some trouble with his/her dress will begin to feel more competent and confident, for it will have at least focused their mind on the importance of the occasion.

Tribunal cases rarely start before 10.00 hours, and as a medical witness, you will be required to be there before the scheduled start time, usually for a last-minute conference especially where barristers or solicitors are representing the parties. The applicant will normally give evidence first. Most tribunals are very sympathetic to the problems that waiting around poses for doctors and will do their best to make specific arrangements to avoid this, often taking the physician, who may be appearing for the respondent, out of turn.

The parties and their witnesses, assemble and wait for the tribunal in separate rooms. The doctor should do the same, but occasionally he may be asked to wait in another room, particularly if jointly instructed by the parties. This practice is increasingly common especially in disability discrimination cases. Under these circumstances, you should not speak to the representatives or the parties, on *either* side, before the case. Nor should you discuss the case with either of the representatives without the other present.

Once you are giving evidence, you are very definitely on your own and you may not, under any circumstances, consult with the other parties in the case. Thus, if you are giving evidence around the time of the lunchtime adjournment, you must expect to take a lonely meal. Isolation begins once the oath has been taken, shortly after taking the stand.

## The witness box

Either the Chair or one of the tribunal wing members will administer the oath. Witnesses will be handed a Bible, usually a New Testament, on the principle that most witnesses are members of the Church of England until proven otherwise. Some tribunals will actually ask your religion and offer you the appropriate religious text. Holders of religious persuasions other than Church of England may require an Old Testament or the Koran, for example. Those who do not follow any religious persuasion may affirm or state in a set form their intention of telling the truth, the consequences of which are identical to those swearing on the Bible.

There is some concern over the appropriateness of the oath to expert witnesses, who give opinions. If you have concerns about this, it is wise to look upon the oath in a somewhat negative fashion. It is an oath that you will not tell an untruth, that you will not deliberately hide a truth and that you will not intentionally answer any question untruthfully. It is, in essence, a public affirmation of the 'expert's declaration' now required under the Civil Procedure Rules and appended to all expert reports.

## Evidence in practice

Questioning usually begins as soon as the oath has been taken. This first stage of evidence is frequently known as the 'examination-in-chief' and brings out the evidence for which you were called to the tribunal. If, for example, you are instructed as a single joint expert, the lead lawyer, who probably instructed you on behalf of the parties, will take you through the report that has already been submitted.

The first role that the representative/lawyer has to do is to introduce the witness to the court. Those introductory questions will require you to give your name, age, address and qualifications. It may be advantageous to be selective. Provided you have the relevant qualifications, there really is no need to rake up the obstetric diploma which you obtained in your youth!

The next phase of giving evidence will place you in relation to the case. It will probably focus on when you were asked to see the applicant by either the applicant or the respondent, or when you received instruction or from whom. Then, it may go on to establish precisely what you were instructed to do.

Next, the evidence will consider what was found. Unless the other party objects, very often the examiner will go directly to the report or statement that was provided to the tribunal and will 'lead the witness'. Once factual matters have been dealt with, opinion evidence will be sought, where appropriate.

Matters of medical knowledge will be brought up and frequently the medical witness – whether the professional or expert – will be asked questions that are strictly outside of their field of competence. This is particularly the case in the lower tribunals. It is tempting to feel some pride in being asked to advise the court on matters relating to neurosurgery or anaesthetics, which would tend to give the impression that, as a physician, you were particularly knowledge-able. True, the tribunal would expect you to have a general, basic knowledge over the range of medicine, but once it involves details of a particular areas about which you do not have special knowledge, you should say so and indicate that you are not competent to express an opinion.

Whenever you *do* express an opinion, however, always attempt to offer the tribunal a range of possibilities, thus preserving your impartiality and your role as an expert witness.

Although the tribunal is not a court of record and a verbatim record is not maintained, the Chair has to maintain a reasonably full record of the proceed-ings, should the decision be challenged before the Employment Appeals Tribunal or similar. Such challenges are likely to increase now that the Human Rights Act 1999 has come into force. Some Chairs have shorthand skills; other type very quickly, but most write longhand. Therefore, when giving your evi-dence, you should watch the Chair's hand, continuing your evidence when it has appeared to stop moving. Equally, if the Chair has embraced information technology, keep an eye on his/her laptop and when his/her fingers are still, move on.

Although it is the lawyer or representative of the parties who asks the questions, it is the tribunal, Chair and wing members who will need to know the answers. Address yourself clearly to the tribunal, calling the Chair 'Sir' or 'Madam'. Speak clearly and loudly enough for the entire tribunal to hear; talk to them directly, especially if the matter is complex. Watch their facial expressions and you will know clearly whether or not your message is getting across.

Consider the general mode of presentation of the evidence. Whilst this is not a court, the Chair and tribunal members will have heard many cases involving medical issues and may well have become familiar with much medical termi-nology. However, it is always good to start off by translating any jargon words that you introduce; and withdraw use if you clearly are causing the tribunal members some annoyance.

In giving evidence, it is important to form a rapport with the tribunal, whether you are appearing as a professional or expert witness. One cannot be condescending; neither can one appear submissive, which will, at best, cast doubts about your expertise and may annoy the tribunal members, who are looking to you for concrete definitive advice. If relations between the you and the tribunal become bad, give some thought to the reason. The expert is not there to usurp the functions of the tribunal. It is not the expert's role to deter-mine whether or not the applicant is 'disabled' within the meaning of the Disability Discrimination Act. That clearly is a question for the tribunal.

Therefore, it is essential that the expert realizes this and does not attempt to take over those functions.

Similarly, a chance request for an opinion is not an opportunity to take over the tribunal's role. Qualifying your comments with, 'This really is a matter for the tribunal,' is not only good common sense, but a cue that gives you a few seconds to think through the reply before offering it to them.

Finally, maintain appropriate forms of address at all times, and resist the temptation to introduce humour, unless it is in response to somebody else's efforts.

## Cross-examination and re-examination

Once the examination-in-chief is completed, it is the turn of the other party to cross-examine. If your evidence is not contentious, there will be no cross-examination; however, depending on the tribunal, cross-examination may be multiple, from different lawyers representing different parties.

The representative or lawyer is required to test the evidence on behalf of his/her client, to make sure that the facts are given accurately, and to probe for any alternative interpretations of the facts more beneficial to their client's case. Cross-examining by the parties in tribunal is given a degree of laxity in the spirit in which the tribunal was formed. As far as employment tribunals are concerned, they were designed to increase access to justice. Cross-examination is given considerable latitude and respondent's witnesses may be in the witness box for several days. This is not an attack upon the witness *per se*, but an effort to cajole an expert witness into modifying their view. It does not happen so much with professional witnesses, who are witnesses of fact.

The cross-examination does nothing more than demonstrate the existence of a doubt; and if important material has been omitted, it is in the interest of *justice*, and not a demonstration of incompetence, that such matters are raised. Hostility from a cross-examining lawyer is only likely to arise when you start prevaricating. Courtesy and consideration normally characterize the cross-examination of an honest witness, be they medical or lay. Fortunately, the coercion of witnesses, by force of rhetoric or character, is long gone and was not usually found in tribunals in any event.

Listen carefully and attentively to the questions posed by the other side. Answer politely and in full. If it is impossible to agree with the proposition that is put to you, politely say so and resist the temptation to attempt to humiliate or be condescending to the questioner, which undoubtedly will fair badly in the eyes of the tribunal.

If you are badgered, resist the temptation to lose your temper, but rather answer firmly, but politely and courteously. The tribunal will have its sympathies with you. If a proposition or idea that has not been considered previously in your evidence is offered, you should take it on board and consider it. You might like to respond that you would like a moment to consider it. The tribunal Chair might even welcome an opportunity for a mid-morning coffee. Whatever you do, resist the temptation to make an ill-considered, snap decision, because introducing such a new proposition opens up opportunities for re-examination.

You must always admit a proposition that is a genuine possibility, although you should state firmly *how* posible you consider the suggestion to be. By the same token, firmly reject any proposal that you consider impossible with explicit reasons for so doing. Such reasons may be very obvious to the doctor, but not necessarily to the tribunal. The opportunity for re-examination, by introducing new material, may be to your advantage, giving you an opportunity to raise your concerns more forcibly. Beware of attempts to manipulate you into supporting a view which does not accord with the actual facts.

Any new material, therefore – including modification of original data – introduced during cross-examination can be re-examined. On re-examination, the lawyer/representative will attempt to counterbalance any points that were conceded in cross-examination. A genuine change of opinion will have to be defended with the same impartiality as was the original, a stance that will require some moral courage. However, re-examination cannot introduce additional new material – it is essentially intended to tidy up the evidence.

Finally, the tribunal Chair or wing members may ask questions to clarify issues to be considered in their own minds. The Chair may interrupt the proceedings at any time during evidence for clarification. Such asides are pertinent and often helpful, even though you may find them disconcerting at the time.

## Conclusions

Doctors giving evidence in tribunals should never lose sight of the fact that their principal duty is to the tribunal and not to those who instructed them. The role of the expert witness is a crucial one within the judicial system, and doctors are accorded privileged positions within the exercise of this role. Tribunals exist to increase access to justice, and in so doing apply legal rules without the strict rules of evidence. This necessarily gives flexibility to those examining witnesses, which is to the advantage of *all* parties.

Tribunals may give the impression of informality but inappropriate and badly presented medical evidence can do much damage to the applicant, the respondent or indeed to the profession. Giving evidence before a tribunal, whether it is a result of joint instructions or of instructions from either of the parties involved, should not be taken on lightly. Every care should be exercised to ensure that the tribunal receives accurate evidence in a manner that they can understand, based on solid foundations and within the context of a strong ethical position. Achieving anything less than the highest professional standards in the giving of evidence will be to the disadvantage of society and to the detriment of our profession.

## Reference

1.  East Lindsey District Council *v* Daubney [1977] IRLR 181

# ▶ 5
# Mental Health Review Tribunals (England and Wales)

The Government has recently published a consultation paper (*Reform of the Mental Health Act, 1983: Proposals for Consultation*, November 1999), which, if carried forward, would make radical changes to the constitution and functions of Mental Health Review Tribunals (MHRTs). It would seem that legislation is unlikely to be enacted in the very near future, so this chapter is geared towards advising psychiatrists who are required to give evidence to MHRTs under the present Act.

MHRTs are independent bodies appointed by the Lord Chancellor to hear appeals against detention, liability to detention or recall, guardianship or supervised discharge in England and Wales. The membership of a tribunal will consist of a lay member and a psychiatrist, and be presided over by a solicitor, barrister or, for restricted cases (section 41), by a circuit judge or QC recorder.

Applications may be made either by the patient or the nearest relative. For patients detained under section 2, applications may be made within 14 days of admission to hospital. For patients detained under section 3 or 37, application may be made within six months of admission to hospital. Patients may be legally represented at hearings. There are also provisions for referral to tribunals by hospital managers and, in restricted cases, by the Home Secretary.

The tribunal will require reports from a social worker and the responsible medical officer (RMO). Although there is no statutory requirement, the tribunal often finds it helpful to have reports from other professionals closely involved in the patient's treatment. It is recognized that hearings can be time-consuming, but, if at all possible, the RMO should be available for at least part of the hearing to give evidence, or, if that is not possible, an experienced junior who has been fully briefed should be available. Medical reports should be clearly dated and, if necessary, updated and be prepared or at least counter-signed by the RMO. Patients usually will be represented by a solicitor or barrister, who may have instructed an independent psychiatrist and/or social worker who may also be called upon to give evidence.

In restricted cases (section 41), the patient may apply to the tribunal for a conditional or absolute discharge. In practice, most discharges are conditional, which may be deferred to allow for specific aftercare arrangements to be made (for example, a hostel placement). Discharge may not be deferred to allow for further observation or treatment as an inpatient. An absolute discharge may be granted either by a tribunal or by the Home Secretary, after the patient has been tested in the community.

*It should be noted that the tribunal is a judicial body and has the power to compel the attendance of witnesses by summons.*

Part V of the Mental Health Act (sections 65–79, of which sections 72 and 73 have particular relevance to RMOs and other psychiatrists who might be called upon to give evidence) deals with tribunals. Although the legal language of the Act itself can be daunting, a study of one of the commentaries on the Act can be helpful. Psychiatric unit libraries would be wise to stock such a publication, and psychiatrists might find that some familiarization with the law can avoid embarrassment at hearings when questioned by members of the panel or the patient's legal representative.

## The hearing

Tribunal hearings are organized by the MHRT regional offices in conjunction with the psychiatric unit Mental Health Act Administrator. Coordinating the attendance of the three panel members, the patient's legal representative, social worker and RMO can be a formidable task. It is therefore helpful if likely problems (including availability due to previous commitments, annual leave, etc.) are communicated as soon as possible after notification of a hearing date.

Apart from those mentioned above, the patient's relatives, a nurse and possibly observers can make for a crowded room, whether in the panelled boardroom of an old psychiatric hospital or a cramped office in one of the newer units, and as such is usually a very stressful experience for the patient. Under the present tribunal rules, the medical member would have seen the patient before the hearing, so that he/she will at least see a familiar face on the other side of the table. Following recent human rights legislation, it has been argued that examination by the medical member might be legally unacceptable, but this has yet to be determined.

The proceedings will be conducted as informally as possible, but the presiding legal member will set the tone and will make sure that each person giving evidence (including the patient) will have his/her say. The hearing is not adversarial; nevertheless, discussion between witnesses and interruptions are not permitted.

The presiding legal member introduces the members but is unlikely to specify the expertise of the 'lay' member. Although lay members may be regarded as representing the general public, they may often have a social work, nursing or other healthcare professional background; they might be a Justice of the Peace or a member of a prison board of visitors and thus be able to ask searching questions.

The RMO (or his/her deputy) is usually the first to give evidence. The panel will have read the medical report (see below) but may need an oral update. The President or medical member will ask the RMO (who, of course, has the authority to discharge in non-restricted cases) to justify continued liability to detention in terms of the statutory criteria set out below:

▶ Is the patient suffering from mental disorder (unspecified for section 2), or mental illness, mental impairment, severe mental impairment or psychopathic disorder in the case of other sections?

▶ Is it currently of a nature or degree that makes it necessary that the patient should remain liable to detention?

▶ Is it necessary for the patient's health, safety, or protection of others?

The panel members will then question in more detail the reason for the RMO's opinion, the treatment being given, future plans and time scale. The tribunal will take into account that hospital care and medication may suppress symptoms and will need to know the likely compliance with treatment should the patient be discharged. Additionally, the tribunal will wish to know whether assessment has been completed in section 2 cases.

The date and conclusions of CPA/section 117 meetings will be of interest to the tribunal. In those cases, where the protection of other persons is an issue, the tribunal will need to know that a risk assessment has been carried out, particularly in restricted cases (section 41). The RMO may recommend a conditional or absolute discharge and will need to convince the tribunal that the criteria for detention are no longer satisfied.

Acting on instructions from his/her client, the patient's representative will question the RMO with a view to demonstrating that the criteria for detention are no longer present. He/she will usually have seen the medical records and may note particularly how often the RMO has assessed the patient and may even seek to cast doubts on the RMO's competence. Fortunately, most legal representatives are sensitive to the fact that it is counterproductive to undermine the doctor–patient relationship, but it is as well to be aware of this possibility.

## The medical report

Reports should be neither too brief nor too loaded with information that is not relevant to the issue of whether the patient should remain liable to further detention.

## Section 2[a]

It is accepted that reports for section 2 tribunals have to be prepared at short notice. Nevertheless, the report needs to contain a brief outline of past history, the reasons for admission for assessment, with progress and treatment (if any) that has been given. The patient's remaining symptoms and mental state should be described in detail and continued detention justified in terms of the statutory criteria.

## Sections 3[b] and 37[c]

Even if patients have had previous tribunal hearings for which medical reports have been prepared, it is unlikely that members of the panel have seen them. A copy of a previous report (clearly dated) may be appended to the current report. All medical reports have to be sent to the tribunal members and the patient's representative (or the patient him/herself, if not represented) and should be prepared as soon as possible after notification of the hearing date, and no later than three weeks before the hearing.

Reports should include a succinct account of:

▶ past history and relevant background, including episodes of self-harm and suicidal ideation

▶ the reasons for admission

▶ symptomatology

▶ treatment and mental state

▶ progress and future plans with reference to CPA and section-117 meetings.

Recommendations should be given, in terms of the statutory criteria, to justify further detention.

## Sections 37[c] and 41[d]

It is particularly important for medical reports to be made available to the regional office in good time, as reports will need to be sent to the Home Office

[a]Section 2 of the Mental Health Act covers admission for re-assessment up to 28 days. [b]Section 3 covers admissions for treatment up to six months (renewable for further periods under s. 20). [c]Section 37 covers admission for treatment imposed by a court on an offender instead of a sentence. [d]Section 41 covers restrictions imposed in addition to s. 37 when a patient has committed a more serious crime (eg homicide, rape, arson or grevious bodily harm). Conditional or absolute discharge may only be granted by the Home Secretary or a tribunal presided over by a judge or QC.

for comment. Failure to do this will preclude the tribunal considering the report and thus lead to an adjournment, which will cause distress to the patient and be a waste of public money.

It is important that the RMO's recommendations for continued detention, deferred conditional, conditional, or absolute discharge should be justified in detail. The tribunal will be particularly interested in the following:

▶ The patient's level of insight into his/her illness and the need for treatment;

▶ Attitude towards the index offence and expressions of remorse or victim empathy (if appropriate);

▶ The patient's behaviour while in hospital, including incidents of unprovoked aggression, compliance with medication, use of occupational facilities and escorted and unescorted leave;

▶ Use and abuse of alcohol and/or illicit drugs.

If conditional discharge is recommended, the tribunal would value the RMO's opinion on appropriate conditions. Although the tribunal's powers are limited to making discharges from the Order, it may make recommendations about leave, transfer, etc., to the Home Office. The comments of the RMO on these issues will be taken into account.

## Bibliography

1. Dolan B, Powell D. *The Mental Health Act Explained*. London: HMSO, 2000
2. Jones R. *Mental Health Act Manual*, 6th edn. London: Sweet and Maxwell, 1999

# ▶6

# The Doctor in the Criminal Court

Doctors may be called upon to give evidence in criminal courts under at least four conditions:

1.  As a witness to fact not linked to any professional activities (eg having witnessed a road accident). In this case, the doctor is a 'lay witness', and the obligations are the same as for any other man or woman in the street.

2.  As a witness to fact relating to a professional matter (eg the examination of a patient). In this case, the doctor is a 'professional witness', bound by professional ethics additional to, but subservient to, the requirements of the law.

3.  As a witness qualified to give an expert opinion on a professional matter in which he has not participated (eg on the medical evidence submitted by the prosecution or defence in a criminal case such as rape or assault). In these cases, the doctor is an 'expert witness'.

4.  As a defendant, for example for an offence under the Road Traffic Act 1991 – or, alas, for manslaughter, having been accused of gross negligence.

The fundamental principle that applies is that information is given to the courts by question and answer. With the exception of the Coroners' court, which will be dealt with elsewhere in this book, you will first be questioned in a criminal court by the lawyer acting for the side which called you, this being the 'examination-in-chief'. You may then be questioned by the other side – 'cross-examination' – which may be followed by 're-examination'. The judge too, may ask you questions directly.

Evidence is given under oath, which will vary according to religious belief, or by affirmation, a form of words which is non-denominational and acceptable to the court. If the witness can be shown not to be telling the truth, a charge of perjury may be laid.

## The professional witness as to fact (1 and 2 above)

You will not be allowed inside the court until called to give evidence. This is to prevent you altering your evidence or opinion subsequent to hearing the evidence of other witnesses.

In a criminal court, commonly you may be a police surgeon (forensic medical examiner), previously called upon to examine a detainee, a law enforcement officer or a victim, or you may be a doctor working in an accident and emergency department. Such evidence will be based upon your written report, referred to as a 'statement', submitted subsequent to your examination of the individual concerned and detailing its findings. The notes you made at the time of the examination, described as 'contemporaneous', may have to be produced for inspection in the court. Where the examinee was in custody, both consent and confidentiality have to be considered. There is recent recognition by the Crown Prosecution Service that doctors giving factual evidence may also give expert evidence in the same case when asked for their opinions. This, however, will not transform the 'professional witness' into an 'expert witness', for the purpose of charging fees.

You may also be called to give evidence about the health of a patient. Again, consent and confidentiality have to be considered.

In any event, absolute impartiality is the rule. The bottom line is that you are there to assist the court, not just the side that instructed you.

## The expert witness (3 above)

Unlike the professional witness, the expert is not only permitted to sit in the court while the case is being heard, but will generally be required to do so by the instructing lawyers. You will listen to the evidence given by other witnesses, compare this with their written statements, and you will advise counsel about matters which fall into your area of expertise in addition to giving your own oral evidence.

In these cases, you will have been asked previously to give an opinion about the findings and opinions of others involved in the case, either directly or indirectly, as in the statement of an expert instructed by the other side. When you are instructed as an expert, it is highly likely that you will have previously been present at a conference involving the solicitors, counsel and any other experts called in to assist them. Submitted statements will be made available to the other side before trial. In court, they are the platform on which oral evidence is built up.

Absolute impartiality is the rule in the preparation of statements and is inherent in the expert's duty to the court. However, when sitting behind counsel and listening to other witnesses, the expert has a duty to the client, either the Crown Prosecution Service or a defendant, to draw counsel's attention to any weakness or flaw in the evidence offered by the other side, adding strength to the side that instructed you. In particular, as stated previously, you will listen carefully to the oral examination of witnesses and relate what is said to what was written previously in statements they have provided and which you should have seen and read. Thus, as an expert witness you may be regarded as having two roles. However, you must remain objective in your advice, and avoid becoming partisan.

## Avoiding pitfalls

### The professional witness

If you are a doctor examining a detainee in a police station or prison, or examining a patient in an accident and emergency department, injured in a road traffic accident or a victim of assault, or simply consulting a patient in primary care, you should be aware that the possibility of subsequent legal involvement. This possibility should always be a major consideration in your documentation of the case and attention to detail at this stage will be most rewarding if you do get so involved.

Giving evidence in court is the final link in a chain of events that has its first link in the understanding of your terms of reference when asked to examine an individual. Any subsequent event, no matter how apparently minuscule at the time, may turn out to be of great importance (for reasons of which you are likely to be unaware) and may form the focus of searching questions when you are in the witness box.

For this reason, your contemporaneous notes are vitally important, so you will be ill-advised to make them in pencil on scrappy pieces of paper. These notes must be given the respect that is demanded of them. Remember that you may be required to produce them in court by order of the judge, and your worth is likely to be assessed in part by their appearance and content.

### *Your notes*

▶ Consider the reasons for making notes

    ▶ To record what you have done, what you have found, the conclusions you have drawn from your findings and anything else you may consider relevant.

▶ To act as an *aide memoire* when you make a statement. If you depart in your statement from the facts recorded in the notes, you will certainly be questioned about the differences. The courts are unlikely to accept that your memory is so good that you can recall *minutiae* absent from your notes months or even years later. To refresh your memory when giving oral evidence in court; but you will require the judge's permission before you refer to your notes. Provided that they were made contemporaneously, or, if that were not possible, at the earliest opportunity thereafter, consent is unlikely to be withheld.

▶ How should notes be kept?

▶ If you are working in an accident or emergency department, you will have to make your notes on the forms provided. Remember that you may be on the other side of the world when the case comes to court, and that someone else, usually the consultant in charge, will have to write a Statement detailing what you have recorded. In all cases, but particularly when your location may change, legibility and a comprehensive approach are vital.

▶ There is a similar situation in primary care. If your notes are made electronically they may be easier to read, but there may be a tendency to abbreviate them as much as possible, the effects of which may make them unintelligible.

▶ Doctors acting as forensic medical examiners will also have forms to complete, but the information given may be inadequate for evidential purposes, so separate contemporaneous notes should be kept. Some doctors prefer to make their notes in hardback A4 books with numbered pages and an integrated index ('minute books'), while others prefer a loose-leaf system. The latter, however, leaves you open to an accusation of substitution.

▶ Write in *ink*, but drawings may be made in pencil.

▶ For reasons that should now be obvious, legibility is a must. The interpretation of a note that is difficult to read may be open to question and may have unwelcome consequences.

▶ When should you make your notes?

▶ As stated above, they should be made at the time of the examination, ie *contemporaneously*. If that is not possible, they should be made *at the earliest time thereafter*. The courts are unlikely to allow you to refer to notes made at other times.

▶ What should your notes contain?

    ▶ If you are using forms supplied by a hospital, for example, you will need to make sure the name of the examinee is correct and that the date and time are given. Recording the gender of the patient is helpful also, particularly when the name is based on a language other than English and it is not self-evident.

    ▶ In other cases, for example as a forensic medical examiner, it is also necessary to ensure that none of these details are omitted.

    ▶ *Consent:* Unless consent is implied, eg by the individual seeking help in an accident and emergency department or in primary care, you will need to obtain *informed* consent to examine. For example, if you are called to examine a detainee, you will need to explain that the ordinary 'rules' of confidentiality may not apply. You should explain that if you become aware of something, eg a health hazard, which should be communicated to the custodians, you have a duty to advise them. Similarly, the detainee should be warned that you might be required to write a Statement and give evidence in court with regard to anything that you observe or become aware of in the course of your examination. Some doctors are content to be given oral consent in the presence of a witness, while others take the view that written consent is desirable. In the former case, your notes should indicate that consent was obtained orally in the presence of a named witness.

    ▶ *History:* The history you take from the examinee should be recorded in detail. In recording information given by the detainee, 'verbals' (ie the actual words used) are often very useful as they impart a flavour of the consultation. If you find any injuries, you should ask how they were received and record the answer. If no answer is given, this too should be recorded. If you have been given information about the examinee, you should state both the information and its source.

    ▶ *The Examination:* If you consider that it is acceptable to limit your examination to a particular anatomical area, you should indicate this and give the reason for it (for example, examination confined to the face in view of an allegation of being punched once on the nose with no other injuries). If a detainee in custody alleges assault by a custodian (eg a police or prison officer), the examination should be comprehensive irrespective of the nature of the allegation. Be methodical. Do not dart about from one system to another. Use classical descriptions since the main readers of this record will be jargon-oriented.

Stick to metric measurements. Record the position, size, shape and colour, and any evidence of healing of injuries. Use body sketches in complicated cases if they are available. It is likely to be relevant to record the examinee's appearance, general behaviour, gait and any odour on the breath. In particular, note any evidence of anxiety, confusion, mental impairment and so on. Above all, record everything you did, everything you found and everything that you expected to find but which was conspicuous by its absence.

▶ *After the examination:* Record the taking of any samples and note their disposal for continuity purposes. Record any advice and/or medication given, and to whom.

## Statements

A request from police for a statement is likely to be the first intimation you will have of your legal involvement in a case. Police will often write statements for lay personnel and get them signed. This is not a practice that should be permitted by the professional. Statements are important documents that may have a wide circulation and they should be treated as such. When you have completed a statement, every page must be signed and checked carefully for errors. Always keep copies.

Statements in criminal cases must be made under section 9 of the Criminal Justice Act 1967 (s.9)*. They must contain this declaration which has to be signed:

> This statement, consisting of x pages each signed by me, is true to the best of my knowledge and belief, and I make it knowing that, if it is tendered in evidence, I shall be liable to prosecution if I have wilfully stated in it anything, which I know to be false or do not believe to be true.

Police may supply printed statement forms, but these are not mandatory. Providing the statement contains the signed declaration described above, it is acceptable.

Statements are best produced on a word processor. Individual templates, specifically created with built-in prompts for this purpose, are valuable time-

---

*Section 9 defines the way in which reports, in England and Wales, may be submitted in criminal cases. In particular, it requires that the author of the statement signs the attestation referred to herein, as well as each page of the report. Having done this, the author is aware that he is liable to prosecution if he contravenes the attestation.

savers and ensure consistency. If they have to be handwritten, it is essential that they are legible.

If any errors are found on checking them, changes must not be made using Tippex or any other correction fluid. The error should be crossed out in ink, and the alteration inserted by hand and initialled.

The statement should contain the following:

▶ Relevant biographical details of your qualifications and experience.

▶ The place and time of the examination.

▶ The identity of the examinee by name and age (and gender if this is not obvious from the name, as is now commonplace in our multicultural, multiracial society).

Never give the address of a victim of assault, sexual or otherwise. Remember the statement has a wide circulation and this address might be communicated to the alleged perpetrator against the wishes of the victim.

In transcribing the findings recorded in your contemporaneous notes, translate medical terms into lay language, since the majority of readers will not be medically literate. An abrasion is a graze, a contusion is a bruise, a laceration is a tear, an incised wound is a cut, the antecubital fossa is the bend of the elbow... and so on.

Explain, with an indication of their significance, medical terms that cannot be translated, eg lateral nystagmus. Include the history given to you by the examinee, but not by third parties (except, of course, parents or carers of young children, for example). In court, if such information from third parties is required, you will be asked in the witness box, and the information may be given by reference to your contemporaneous notes. Be *precise*, *concise* and *unbiased*.

Never write anything in a statement that you cannot substantiate in the witness box in the face of vigorous cross-examination.

## The expert witness

At present, it is for the courts to decide whether or not you are acceptable to give evidence as an expert. Their assessment will be based on your qualifications and experience. However, the Council for the Registration of Forensic Practitioners (CRFP) has recently been established with the support of the Home Office, in order 'to create, maintain and promote public confidence in forensic practice'. It proposes to do this by publishing a register of competent practitioners, by ensuring through periodic revalidation, that forensic practitioners keep up to date and maintain competence, and by dealing with registered practitioners who fail to meet the necessary standards. Registration of doctors working in the criminal area of the medico-legal interface will be invited shortly. Failure to be registered with the CRFP may well become disadvantageous to the expert in court.

Doctors wishing to undertake work as an expert witness are strongly advised to join one of the organisations offering help to the expert and these are listed in Appendix 1. Training in the writing of expert reports (in s.9 format) is available, as are courses on courtroom skills.

The general rule is that the expert witness will have had no contact with the parties in the case and will be giving opinion evidence rather than factual evidence. However, there are regional differences. In Manchester, for example, doctors working in a sexual assault centre are paid by the courts as experts even though they have been directly involved in the examination of a victim and are giving evidence as to fact. Their colleagues in the Metropolitan Police area are often not so fortunate.

## The sequence of events

### 1. The initial approach

If you have indicated your willingness to undertake this work and have either been included in one or more of the expert witness registers or have been recommended personally, defence lawyers seeking assistance will probably telephone you to see if you are willing and available. You should ask for a brief outline of the case to assess whether or not it lies within your area of expertise. If it does not, say so and recommend a suitable colleague if you know of one. *Never* accept instructions when the case is outside your area of expertise.

The lawyer will want to know your likely fee for providing a report. Hourly rates payable by the Legal Services Commission (LSC) are published, but estimating the amount of time preparing a report will take is an art in itself. It depends very much on the size of the file that you are going to have to read, how well the lawyers have prepared it, how much research of the literature will be required, and, of course, the speed at which you work.

They will also want to know how quickly you can provide the report. Even more importantly, a date may already have been set for trial, and if you are not going to be available, there is no point in going any further.

### 2. Your response

If the case is one that you feel competent to undertake and you are available within the lawyer's time constraints, you should say so and suggest a fee that will not exceed £x. This will be put to the LSC for approval, if this applies. Whilst this is being done, you should send the lawyers a letter indicating your willingness to help, quoting the estimate and the time scale. Your CV should accompany the letter. If the case is funded privately, agreement may be reached directly. In these cases, you will be asked to give your daily rate for attendance at Court. There have been problems regarding delayed payment of fees in publicly funded cases. In any event, model contracts and/or terms of agreement are available from the helping organizations, and their use is recommended. You should also ask to see the authority for your fee provided to the instructing solicitor by the LSC, for this prior authority guarantees payment. The LSC will pay experts' fees by disbursements, so delays should be avoidable.

The next stage is for the lawyers to send you the case file. This should contain all the documents you will need. In cases of assault, sexual or otherwise, these should include the indictment, statements by the complainant, other witnesses and police officers, medical reports, and statements by the defendant.

## 3. The case file

This should have been prepared by the lawyers and contain all the relevant documentation, which should be indexed. S.9 statements by doctors who have examined the individual(s) concerned should be accompanied by copies of the doctor's contemporaneous notes. If they are not included in the bundle, you should advise the lawyers that they must be obtained. You must be able to compare their contemporaneous notes with their statements, and, in due course, with their oral evidence. It is up to you to ensure that all the relevant documents are available for your perusal.

## 4. Your investigation

The entire file will need to be read and you should bear this in mind when estimating your fee. Your approach should be methodical; for example, if you have been instructed by defence, in an assault case – sexual or otherwise – a logical approach would be as follows:

- Consider the indictment.
- Look at s.9 statements by the complainant and any supporting witnesses. Any photographs should be viewed.
- List the alleged physical contacts.

▶ Look at the contemporaneous notes and any s.9 statements by the examining doctors and consider their opinions.

▶ Look at any s.9 statement by the defendant and any supporting s.9 statements.

▶ If the defendant has been examined medically, look at the contemporaneous notes and s.9 statements of the doctors, and consider their opinions.

▶ Relate the allegation to the medical findings and consider the validity of the medical opinions offered by the prosecution.

▶ Where there is a range of opinion, particularly in sexual assault cases, review the literature and consider your own opinion carefully.

## 5. Your report and opinion

Generally, in criminal cases the instructing lawyer will ask you to prepare the report in s.9 format. It should contain your qualifications, relevant biographical details and highlight your training in the specialized area. Counsel will lead you through this in order to demonstrate to the jury that your opinion is one that should be respected. It is not an ego trip, so it is important that it is comprehensive and not diminished by modesty.

You should also state your instructions and list the documents with which you have been provided.

Deal with each stage of your investigation, numbering them sequentially. Within each section, it is useful to number each sentence. Double-spacing is appreciated by the lawyers, who can make annotations on copies in due course.

The final section of your report is your opinion. Individual opinions should be related numerically to the investigatory sections.

If you agree with any part of the medical evidence offered by the other side of the adversarial contest, you should say so; otherwise, your report would be suspected of bias. Areas of disagreement should be clearly defined and your reasons given, supported by references where this would be helpful. The references should be included in the report as an appendix.

In the civil area, medical experts are already required to add an expert's declaration to their reports. Although it is currently neither mandatory nor common practice, in criminal cases this can be adapted and usefully added to the end of a s.9 statement thus:

> I understand that my overriding duty is to the court, both in preparing statements and in giving oral evidence.
> I have set out in my statement what I understand from those

instructing me to be the questions in respect of which my opinion as an expert are required.

I have done my best, in preparing this statement, to be accurate and complete. I have mentioned all matters that I regard as relevant to the opinions I have expressed. All of the matters on which I have expressed an opinion lie within my field of expertise.

I have drawn to the attention of the court all matters of which I am aware that might adversely affect my opinion.

Wherever I have no personal knowledge, I have indicated the source of factual information.

I have not included anything in this statement which has been suggested to me by anyone, including the lawyers instructing me, without forming my own independent view of the matter.

Where, in my view, there is a range of reasonable opinion, I have indicated the extent of that range in the statement.

At the time of signing the statement, I consider it to be complete and accurate. I will notify those instructing me if, for any reason, I subsequently consider that the statement requires any correction or qualification.

I understand that this statement will be the evidence that I will give under oath, subject to any correction or qualification I may make before swearing to its veracity.

I believe that the facts I have stated in this statement are true and that the opinions I have expressed are correct.

**(Adapted from the Expert Witness Declaration, issued by the EWI)**

## Submission of your statement

Having submitted your statement, you may be approached by the lawyers to include or exclude an item. Whether or not you comply is a matter for your mature judgement, bearing in mind that your primary duty is to the court.

## Going to court

Once it is decided that your presence in court is necessary and a date has been fixed, if you are instructed by defence, some lawyers will serve you with a Witness Summons (formerly a Subpoena). The purpose of this is to prevent your involvement with other cases interfering with your ability to attend. Having said that, it is not unknown for date and/or time of your appearance to be altered at the last moment. It can be very frustrating and a source of considerable irritability. However, it may be somewhat mollified by the possibility of claiming cancellation fees (provided these have been included in your agreement with the instructing solicitor beforehand).

## The court appearance

### *Magistrates' Courts*

Professional witnesses are often required to give oral evidence in Magistrates' Courts. These tend to be very busy places and their procedures are less formal than in the higher courts. The court may be presided over by a Stipendiary Magistrate or by a Justice of the Peace sitting with two colleagues. Either way, as in all courts, make sure you use the correct title for the magistrate, Sir or Madam is usually appropriate. You will be called to give your evidence, but will not be permitted to sit in the court beforehand, unlike the expert witness.

### *Crown courts*

These courts are much more formal, with tighter controls over procedure. Once again, the professional witness will not be permitted to sit in the court until called to give evidence, whereas the expert witness will need to be in court to hear the oral evidence. Rules of conduct in court are common to all witnesses. There is one particular feature, however, of which the tyro witness should be very aware. Having been sworn or affirmed as the case may be, you will be asked questions about your involvement in the case. You will have brought with you all the documents you need, but you may not refer to any of them without the permission of the court. You should address the judge, using his or her correct title – Your Honour or My Lord – and ask if you may refer to your notes to refresh your memory. The judge will ask when you made those notes, and you should reassure the court that they were made contemporaneously. Permission will be granted.

## Hints and tips

▶ *Timekeeping:* You will have been given a time to attend court. Although it is highly likely that you will have to wait, you should not be late. If you are unavoidably detained – which does happen – notify the court by telephone as soon as possible.

▶ *Dress:* Dress professionally. Your appearance *does* matter – juries and judges are not impressed by T-shirts and jeans. However, the following story has a message:

*A judge sitting in a Crown Court was much vexed by the lateness of a medical witness. When the doctor did finally arrive, he was dressed in a crumpled T-shirt and jeans, with a fresh growth of facial stubble and looking most unkempt. The judge was just about to tear him off a strip when the doctor addressed him. 'Your Honour,' he said, 'Forgive my lateness and appearance. I have been on duty in my accident and emergency department for the last eighteen hours and I have had no time to change or clean myself up. Please be assured that I mean no disrespect to the Court.'*

The judge told this story at the Royal Society of Medicine (London, UK) subsequently, and said that from that moment that particular witness could not put a foot wrong.

▶ *Demeanour:*

- ▶ Make sure your mobile phone is turned off.

- ▶ Remember that you are there to assist the court, so avoid being partisan.

- ▶ Your evidence must be heard, so speak up.

- ▶ It helps to base your stance in the direction of the judge. In this way, although you will look at counsel when being asked questions, your body will swing towards the judge when you reply, for it is to the judge (and jury) that your replies should be addressed.

- ▶ Your answers should be as concise and precise as possible.

- ▶ Do not volunteer information. If you do, you may find yourself in deep water.

- ▶ Beware the 'Yes, but...' response. The 'Yes' indicates agreement, which may not be appropriate. It is safer to say, 'I hear what you say, but...'

- ▶ You are not omniscient and cannot be expected to be so. If you are asked a question to which you do not know the answer, say so and make no attempt to waffle.

- ▶ If you are asked a question outside your area of expertise, say so, and suggest the discipline to which the question should be put.

- ▶ Never lose your temper – you might be provoked in the hope that you will do so. Try very hard not to allow any irritation which you may feel to show in your face, voice or body language.

- ▶ It is most unwise to be flippant with counsel or, in particular, with the judge. The witness box can suddenly become a lonely place.

▶ When your evidence has been heard and there are no more questions to be put, ask the judge if you may be released.

▶ Don't leave the court without a form on which to claim your fee.

## The expert witness

Sitting behind counsel, you will listen to the evidence and draw counsel's attention to matters about which you are competent to opine. This may be done by handing him clearly written concise messages, not on scraps of paper, but on pages of at least A5 size. This is particularly important when counsel is engaged in cross-examination.

Although it has become common in civil cases for the court to instruct experts to confer in order to reach agreement and/or define differences of opinion, this has not been common in criminal cases. However, there is little doubt that this is now happening, since it saves considerable time and expense. There should be an agreed agenda. Whether or not lawyers should be present at meetings of experts is arguable.

## The future

At the end of 1999, the Lord Chancellor, Lord Irvine of Lairg, appointed the Rt. Hon. Lord Justice Auld, to review and report on the working of the criminal courts. His terms of reference were as follows:

> Review into the practices and procedures of, and the rules of evidence applied by, the criminal courts at every level, with a view to ensuring that they deliver justice fairly, by streamlining all their processes, increasing their efficiency and strengthening the effectiveness of their relationships with others across the whole of the criminal justice system, and having regard to the interests of all parties, including victims and witnesses, thereby promoting public confidence in the rule of law.

At the time of writing, he had not yet reported. Clearly, his report is likely to have as much effect on the criminal justice system as the Woolf Report has had for reforming civil procedure and rules.

## Reference

1. *Access to Justice*. The Final Report of the Right Honourable Lord Woolf. London: HMSO, July 1996

# ▶7
# The Doctor and the Civil Courts

## Introduction

A doctor may be called to give evidence before civil courts as:

▶ a defendant

▶ a lay witness

▶ an expert witness.

The role of the doctor as defendant in a medical negligence action is addressed elsewhere in this book (Chapter 2) and shall not be dealt with here.

## The doctor as lay witness

In the context of a clinical negligence case, doctors and other healthcare professionals involved in the claimant's care may be called upon to give evidence of *fact* for either claimant or defendant. The first intimations that a complaint is to be made come in a letter from the claimant's legal advisers, the 'letter of claim'. In a protocol published by the Lord Chancellor's Department[1] in July 1998, it is stressed that, in all specialties, healthcare providers should, at an early stage, set up adverse outcome reporting systems so that statements can be obtained from key witnesses. Therefore, once a letter of claim has been received, these statements are available for review and, if necessary, amplification. The defendant doctor or Trust has three months in which to prepare a *reasoned answer.*[1]

If the matter proceeds to the issue of a claim form, the claimant must then set out before the court a formal statement, the *particulars of claim*. Within a specified but relatively short period, the defendant must answer the particulars of claim with a 'defence'. These documents are now called 'statements of case', formally known as pleadings. Each has now to be accompanied by a statement of truth, and no evidence can be given that does not relate to the allegations therein. Once the defence has been served, there may be an opportunity for clarification of the issues through requests for the provision of further information. A procedural judge will then allocate the case to a track and give directions for the management of the case, in the first instance by fixing a case-management conference at which a timetable for the action will be set. The judge will issue an order limiting the number of experts to be called. The timetable will usually require the mutual simultaneous exchange of lay witness evidence, followed, after a period of a few weeks, by the simultaneous exchange of expert evidence.

On the claimant's side, the lay evidence usually will be from the claimant and perhaps a close relative; occasionally, it will include statements from an ambulance driver, nurse or other healthcare worker. On the defendant's side, all those healthcare practitioners who were involved in the claimant's treatment will usually be required to provide statements and, if necessary, to give evidence in court. Occasionally, the claimant may call a doctor, nurse or midwife involved in the treatment who, for whatever reason, has not been called by the defence.

In principle, these witnesses are no different from witnesses of fact called in other courts of law. They have the same obligation to tell the truth and are afforded the same protection against civil suit. There is the important difference, however, that in calling a doctor to give factual evidence about a medical matter, a court may come to rely upon the doctor's special knowledge and understanding of the events at the centre of the dispute. It may be necessary for the doctor, in giving his factual evidence, to interpret specialist terminology or explain certain medical procedures to the court. Explanation fades imperceptibly into opinion and so the lay witness called to give factual evidence will inevitably, from time to time, be drawn into giving opinion (expert) evidence to the court.

Greater flexibility of procedure in professional negligence trials has tended to exacerbate this problem. In the old days, when the claimant's case was heard in its entirety before any evidence was called for the defendant, there was the opportunity for the claimant's expert to 'explain' all the difficult and contentious matters to the judge and to give his/her opinion evidence alongside it. Now (unless counsel explains the technical matters in the skeleton argument), when factual evidence is called first, the court has its first opportunity to hear about complex medical matters in the course of the evidence of lay witnesses. This leads to 'expert evidence' inevitably being given by doctors and other healthcare professionals because without it the court cannot understand their factual evidence. Provided the explanation is uncontentious, there need be no objection to this procedure, but there is always the temptation for the experienced senior doctor giving factual evidence early in a case to put a sufficient 'spin' on the explanatory aspects of his evidence as to make him, effectively, an expert.

In the present climate, procedural judges are keen to restrict the number of experts called by each side and they impose increasingly frugal limits on the parties. The defendant who introduces a senior doctor, and often more than one, early in the case can effectively circumvent this limit by using lay witnesses as experts. In my experience, it is not uncommon for a statement to be served from the named consultant under whose care the claimant was admitted to hospital but who will say in their statement that he/she never met the claimant. The doctor is, of course, witness to nothing, just another senior doctor able to give opinion evidence under the guise of a lay witness. To correct this imbalance, the claimant may get an order from the court that witness statements shall not contain opinion evidence, and may later be able to have any opinion evidence struck out.

## The report

The key to successful defence of unmeritorious negligence actions is *early*, *accurate*, *thorough* and *honest* clinical incident reporting.

As part of the risk management process,[2,3] all members of staff associated with an adverse outcome are required to produce factual reports at the earliest possible opportunity. The report is compiled when memory is fresh and with the assistance of the patient's clinical records. The simple guidelines for the construction of such reports are given in Box 7.1.

Your initial report must be factual. It must not contain opinion nor seek to apportion blame. It should reconstruct, as accurately as possible, the circumstances obtaining at the time, the personnel involved and the timing of events.

| Box 7.1. | |
|---|---|
| **The report should never:** | **The report should:** |
| a) Be hastily compiled. | a) Be totally honest. |
| b) Be brief and dismissive. | b) Be thorough and exhaustive. |
| c) Seek to blame others for what happened. | c) Deal with what can *actually* be remembered. |
| d) Go beyond personal knowledge and recollection. | d) Reconstruct the clinical thinking considerations and options in the minds of the doctor at the time. |
| e) Be concerned with the aftermath, rather than the incident. | e) Concentrate on what *was* done rather than what *would have* been done. |
| f) Include irrelevant subjective comments about the patient or others. | f) Include, as far as possible, details of time and the identity of personnel. |

There is often confusion in hospital notes concerning the times recorded. Should the time recorded be taken to indicate the time of the event or simply the time when the note was written? A statement made within a few days of the event may be helpful in clarifying such issues.

The report so generated will form the basis of the evidence you will give to a court, should the matter come to trial. It is unlikely that, at a later stage, details of the reconstruction can honestly be added, for memory inevitably fades. It may be appropriate at a later stage, however, to amplify those sections of the report which relate to protocol and procedure, filling in the gaps which inevitably remain with an honest assessment of what 'would have been done' in accordance with normal practice.

Sadly, many medical reports submitted as lay witness evidence are written entirely in the subjunctive and deal only with 'what would have been done', for no one has thought to ask the doctor to record the events sufficiently close to the time of the incident. Such reports inevitably carry less weight than those written with clear recollection and made within a few hours or days of the adverse outcome.

## Oral evidence

When you are giving factual witness evidence, the witness box should hold few fears, provided you stick to an honest rehearsal of the facts. Be modest, succinct and intelligible. Usually called by the defendant, you will be expected to answer questions under cross-examination from the claimant's counsel. The timing and sequence of events will often be challenged. It is essential that, in such circumstances, you go no further then you can honestly remember, aided by the report you wrote at the time. You may be asked to supply details you cannot honestly remember; where memory runs out, you should say so and avoid the temptation of helpful creativity. You may be caught out and that part of your evidence honestly remembered then will no longer be believed.

### The doctor as expert

Since at least the 16th century, the courts have called upon scientists to explain matters that are beyond the knowledge of the ordinary man in the street.[4] Expert knowledge was often found amongst the jury; the expert witness, called before the court to give both explanatory evidence and opinion, dates from the 18th century. In 1782, Lord Mansfield[5] allowed the opinion evidence of a famous engineer, Mr Smeaton, as to whether the erection of a bank had caused the silting up of a harbour:

> ... in matters of science, the reasonings of men of science can only be answered by men of science... It is objected that Mr. Smeaton is going to speak, not of the facts, but as to opinion. That opinion, however, is deduced from the facts which are not disputed... I cannot believe that where the question is, whether a defect arises from a natural or an artificial cause, the opinions of men of science are not to be received.

In *medical negligence* cases, experts are required to assist the court in determining issues both of liability and quantum (see Box 7.2).

---

**Box 7.2.** *Experts are required to assist the court in:*

**Liability**
- ▶ Breach of duty
- ▶ Causation

**Quantum**
- ▶ Extent of injury
- ▶ Present condition
- ▶ Prognosis
- ▶ Future treatment
- ▶ Future needs for care.

---

The existence of the duty of care is seldom in dispute; the *discharge* of that duty is the critical issue in negligence, and the expert is required to establish the appropriate standard of care at the time, and the extent to which that duty of care was achieved.

The standards appropriate are those obtaining at the time of the incident. Not so with issues of causation. In determining whether an alleged breach of duty led to the claimant's injuries, the court will be concerned to hear the best information available – the most up-to-date and modern opinion about causation, not the state of the art as it was when the injury occurred.

Quantum experts are, of course, drawn from many different professions as well as medicine and will include architects, surveyors, engineers, occupational therapists and other healthcare professionals.

In other types of *personal injury* cases, the duty and its breach are seldom matters for medical comment. The doctor in such cases is concerned with causation and quantum, assisting the court to understand the relationship between the accident and the victim's present condition.

Most of what follows relates specifically to the role of the expert in *medical negligence* litigation. In this context, expert evidence is much more contentious because the expert is required to assess and evaluate the conduct of his peers and to give his opinion on matters concerning medical competence. In personal injury litigation, medical evidence is, in my experience, seldom called and can usually be agreed after negotiation. Whilst oral evidence in medical negligence is still not common, it occurs, at least in my practice, in about 5% of the cases in which I am instructed.

## The role of the expert: as witness and as adviser

When approached initially by either claimant or defendant, the expert must be – and must be seen to be – truly independent. He/she should have no connection with either party and should give his/her opinion in a dispassionate and disinterested manner. It may be that, having formed an opinion, the expert advises the party that he cannot support the case. In such circumstances, that is usually the end of the matter. If, however, you, as expert, find yourself able to support the case for claimant or defendant, that case inevitably will be based on your opinion. In an adversarial system, you, as expert, necessarily become part of the legal team and will be expected to advise on the conduct of the case, not only in the presentation of expert evidence for your 'side' but also in challenging the evidence produced by experts on the other side.

There is a tension between the roles; both experts *and* lawyers often have difficulty in understanding their proper limits. Much has been written about the duties of the expert as witness by Lord Wilberforce in *Whitehouse v Jordan*,[6] by Cresswell J. in the *Ikarian Reefer*,[7] by Lord Woolf in *Access to Justice*,[8] and in the New Civil Procedure Rules (CPR) Part 35 (see Appendix 7.1 below).[9] Little has been written about the role of the expert as adviser – a role best understood by following the process of a claim.

## Training

Doctors often are inclined to believe that they have only to use their ordinary medical skills in order to be satisfactory expert witnesses. At present, however, the medical curriculum contains almost no law, and certainly no training in this field. When first approached, a doctor may have little idea of what is required of him by the courts in providing expert evidence. Training therefore is essential. It does not follow that because a doctor is experienced in his profession and eminent in his field he will necessarily make a satisfactory expert witness. To do that, he must have some understanding of what the courts require.

When I began giving expert evidence in 1970, there was no training. Along with others of my generation, I learnt by making my own mistakes, often at the expense of the public purse. Experts, ignorant of the law within which they operate, are a menace to the courts for they waste time, addressing the wrong questions and applying the wrong standards. There is no longer any excuse for this – there is ample training available for those who wish to avail themselves of it. The Expert Witness Institute (see Appendix 1 for details) runs a full training programme, including a course in basic law for experts. In providing such education, the Institute was responding to the challenge laid down by Lord Woolf in *Access to Justice*:[10]

> I certainly support the provision of training for experts, both through attendance at courses and through the dissemination of published material... Professional people who take on responsibilities as expert witnesses need a basic understanding of the legal system and their role within it. They also need to be able to present their evidence effectively, both in written reports and orally under cross-examination. Training in presentational skills, however, should never lose sight of the fundamental point that the expert's duty is to assist the court. Otherwise it is not in the interests of justice because it may result in the truth being concealed.

In order to be effective, an expert must understand the essential elements of procedure as set out in the CPR.

## Procedure

1.  Pre-action
    ▶ Investigation
    ▶ Letter of claim
    ▶ Disclosure.
2.  Instruction of experts.
3.  The expert report.
4.  Conference.
5.  Statements of case.
6.  Experts discussion.
7.  Oral evidence.

## Pre-action

Figure 7.1, an annexe to the Pre-action Protocol,[1] illustrates the likely sequence of events of a clinical dispute.

At stage d (or even earlier), good clinical governance[11] requires an appraisal of the clinical incident by an inhouse expert. A consultant of the appropriate specialty employed by the Trust or Health Authority will provide an overview that can be used in the initial stages to guide the response of the provider unit to the complaint. Such a procedure has the merit of being both fast and free but the expert so instructed will never become a witness for he is not truly 'independent', being an employee of the provider unit. His role is only that of *adviser*.

The claimant, on the other hand, at stage D, instructs an independent expert. The defendant's first independent expert may not be instructed until after the issue of proceedings.

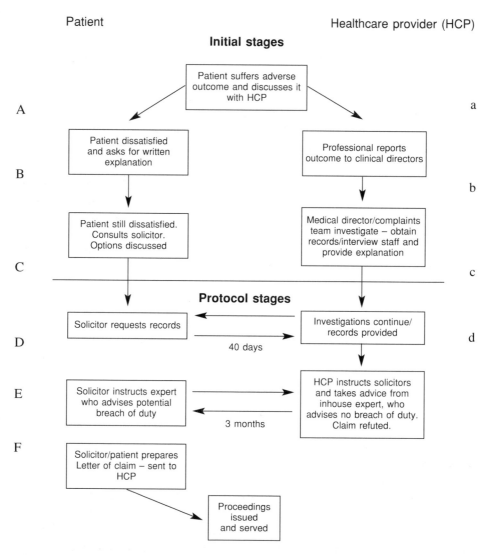

**Fig. 7.1.** *The likely series of events of a clinical dispute: an illustrative flowchart*

# The instruction of the claimant expert

The essential requisites of the expert witness on liability are illustrated in Box 7.3.

| **Box 7.3.** *The qualities of an expert witness* |
|---|
| ▶ Independent |
| ▶ Of appropriate speciality |
|    ▶ in comparable practice at the time |
|    ▶ still in active practice (if possible) |
| ▶ Trained in the duties of an expert |

It is not always possible to obtain an expert who was in the appropriate practice at the time of the clinical event and who is still in current active practice. Some stale claims relating to birth injury are brought *20 or more years* after the event and practitioners familiar with the standards of practice at the time may no longer be active clinically. The essential pre-requisite is an understanding of the clinical standards relevant at the time of the incident.

To be independent, the expert must not be a treating doctor and must not be — professionally or personally — closely associated with the defendant. He also must have an independence of attitude that allows him to approach such problems with an open mind and without prejudice in favour of either defendant or claimant. The striking of attitudes by expert witnesses in favour of either claimant or (more usually) defendant has seriously undermined the credibility of medical expert witnesses. The polarization of experts was the subject of adverse comment from Lord Woolf in *Access to Justice*.[12]

As an expert, you should not be tempted to stray outside you own particular field of expertise. It is common for specialists to comment on the standard provided by general practitioners, midwives and nurses, but the standards for each healthcare professional should be set by their peers, for only *they* have first-hand experience of the issues before the court.

The choice of an appropriate expert may present formidable difficulties to the inexperienced claimant solicitor. There are published lists of experts willing to take on cases; some of the Royal Colleges produce lists of 'volunteers' but cannot speak to their experience or training as expert witnesses. Both the Academy of Experts and the Expert Witness Institute keep lists of doctors by speciality. Whilst membership of one of these organizations indicates some training (or at least a willingness to take part in training programmes), these bodies are not yet able to match experts with cases. The best source of advice for claimant solicitors remains AVMA (Action for the Victims of Medical Accidents), who maintain not only a comprehensive list of experts but also a trained staff willing and able to advise on selection for a particular case.

The selection of a suitable expert for the defence creates less difficulty for a number of reasons. Medical defence organizations have their own lists of tried and tested experts; most medical defence is now handled by relatively few firms of solicitors and they too have their own lists. The doctors concerned will usually know – by reputation – of suitable experts in the field.

Once selected, the expert needs to be instructed. Before a full letter of instruction, the wise solicitor will write a preliminary letter setting out:

▶ the identity of the defendant

▶ the identity of the individual treating doctor(s)

▶ the name of the claimant

▶ the date of the clinical incident

▶ the broad nature of the event, the nature of the complaint and the damages suffered.

Only then can the expert indicate whether a possible conflict of interest might arise or whether the nature of the accident and the circumstances of its occurrence lie within their field of expertise. This exchange of correspondence will enable the expert to inform the solicitor of:

▶ the waiting list

▶ the cost of the report

▶ the terms of engagement.

It is important to establish at the outset the terms under which the expert is prepared to act. Under the CPR (35.4),[9] the courts may not only restrict the number of experts who can be *called* but also may control the level of fees:

> The court may limit the amount of the expert's fees and expenses that the party who wishes to rely on the expert may recover from any other party.
>
> **CPR 35.4(4)**

Thus, the cost of the report agreed at the beginning may not be recoverable by the instructing party at the end of the case, should they win. The solicitor may seek at the beginning an undertaking from the expert that he will agree to repay, or waive, part of his fee if the court restricts recovery. If the expert is not prepared to accept such conditions, he must say so at the outset, before incurring any costs or undertaking any work.

Once agreed in principle, the solicitor will formally instruct the expert (see Box 7.4).

---

**Box 7.4.** *Instruction to the claimant expert*

---

- ▶ A brief summary of clinical events
- ▶ Injuries suffered by the claimant
- ▶ Copy of correspondence with the defendants
- ▶ A full legible set of indexed, paginated medical records
- ▶ A list of other experts instructed
- ▶ The claimant's witness statement
- ▶ Any other relevant witness statements
- ▶ Identification of the issues in the case.

---

The quality of instructions from the claimant's solicitor varies enormously, and some are no better than the legendary general practitioner reference to the specialist 'please see and advise'. If the case is worth funding (either by public funding from the Legal Services Commission or by conditional fee), the solicitor should be aware of the issues to be addressed by the expert and these should be clearly set out in the letter of instruction. The CPR (Part 35.10[3])[9] require the expert, in the report he produces to the court, to state 'the substance of all material instructions, whether written or oral, on the basis of which the report was written'.

The experienced claimant solicitor will have a clear idea, from the beginning, of the number of specialties in which expert opinion is required and the identities of those experts. In other cases, it may be appropriate to use the main liability expert as the 'lead expert', around whom the claimant team is built. There is much to be said for using experts who are used to working together.

## The instruction of the defendant expert

Formal instruction of an independent expert for the defence does not usually occur until after proceedings have been issued. In general, the quality of instruction from defendant solicitors has been of better quality because the work is concentrated into fewer firms and most defendant work is in the hands of specialists. Surprisingly, statements from key healthcare providers are often missing. It is, of course, essential for the defendant expert to see statements from all the treating clinicians, as well as any guidelines or protocols in use within the unit at the time. Ideally, the defendant expert should be able to meet the key clinicians before preparing his report, but one finds that one is seldom permitted to do so; one usually meets them – if at all – only in conference, discovering, perhaps for the first time, their decision-making process which led to the incident in question.

---

**Box 7.5.**   *Instruction to the defendant expert*

---

- ► Brief summary of clinical events
- ► Injury suffered by the claimant
- ► Copy of the letter of claim and other correspondence with the claimant
- ► A full legible set of medical records
- ► List of other experts instructed
- ► Witness statements from all of the healthcare professionals involved
- ► Identification of the issues in the case

---

If there have been preliminary inhouse views on liability, you should expect to see them.

## Privilege

Since introduction of the CPR, there has been considerable confusion, doubt and concern about how much of what an expert says or writes must be disclosed to the other side, apart from the formal report to the court. Part 35 is not clear in this regard. Adrian Whitfield QC[13] has helpfully reviewed the subject and advises the following:

- ► Pre-litigation reports by an expert need not be disclosed[14]

- ► Post-litigation advice by an expert, unless it indicates a change of view, is *advice* to the client and need not be disclosed.

- ► Instructions to experts remain privileged save only for the circumstances outlined in CPR 35.10.

CPR 35.10(3) requires the expert to 'state the substance of all material instructions, whether written or oral, on the basis of which the report was written'. The difficulty for the expert is the next paragraph (35.10[4]):

> The instructions referred to in paragraph (3) shall not be privileged against disclosure but the court will not, in relation to those instructions –
> (a) order disclosure of any specific document; or
> (b) permit any questioning in  court, other than by the party who instructed the expert,
> unless it is satisfied that there are reasonable grounds to consider the statement of instructions given under paragraph (3) to be inaccurate or incomplete.

As far as I am aware, this provision has not been tested in a court, and experts remain confused about just how much detail of their instructions the court expects to be included in this statement.

Where the expert, having written a report or having given evidence in court, changes his view, that change of view must be communicated to the court at the earliest opportunity.

## The medical records

It is not part of your duty as an expert to obtain the medical records; that privilege belongs to the parties' legal advisers. It is your duty, however, to advise the lawyers when disclosure of medical records is inadequate or incomplete.

Whether instructed by claimant or defendant, it is essential that you see *all* of the medical records. This will usually mean the general practitioner records as well as those dealing with any hospital admission. It will also mean seeing the notes of related hospital admissions, perhaps in different hospitals. In obstetric cases, it is almost always necessary to see the notes of *all* pregnancies, not just that about which complaint is made. The quality standards for the provision of medical records are set out in annexe B to the Pre-action Protocol for resolution of clinical disputes.[1] You should not accept incomplete or illegible records. If vital passages are illegible, you should advise the instructing solicitor to request a transcript by the author – or at least inspection of the original. You should not accept records reproduced in other than their original format. Charts (such as those produced in intensive care units, or partograms) which originated as A3 documents should be so reproduced. Long records of electronic recording should be reproduced in continuous rolls and not chopped up into A4 or A3 segments. Although the mechanism for producing such records[15] has been advertized widely since 1990, it is nevertheless the common experience of experts that the advice is not followed. Satisfactory copies of long documents such as cardiotocograph traces (CTGs) can often be made by feeding the original through an old-fashioned domestic fax machine. Professional copies can be obtained from *The Times* Drawing Office, 15 Maddox Street, London W1 (Tel: 020 7629 7500).

Unless you have a full and complete set of hospital records, you cannot be expected to assess care appropriately. The assessment of records is greatly improved if they are organized, indexed and paginated. Experienced firms of solicitors often will perform this task inhouse. Others use professional note-sorting agencies, some of whom perform the task distinctly better than others. Several of the organizations with grand sounding names do an appalling job and are not worth the fee. In my experience, the best in the field are:

▶ Ms Helen Doig, 5 Mawddach Crescent, Arthog, Gwynedd LL39 1BJ.
  Tel: 01341 250 599; Dx: 711442 Dolgellau

*and*

▶ Dr A Roderick MBBS (Lond), 6 Sway Road, Morriston, Swansea
  SA6 6HT. Tel: 01792 701 681.

However it is done, it is a great advantage to everyone, not only the expert. In reconstructing the events of the incident in question you will need to quote from the medical records, indicating the appropriate page. Unless the pages are numbered, this task is impossible. Certainly, if the matter ever comes before a court, counsel will need a quick reference to the page numbers in dealing with the expert report in evidence.

Every page of the hospital records should be examined. The nursing records are of particular importance since frequently they give critical insight into the timing of medical intervention and the reasons for it. Nurses, in general, keep better notes than doctors, are more scrupulous about time and invaluably refer to the names of doctors whose signatures may be illegible. General practitioner records often contain important correspondence not produced in the hospital records.

It is surprising how often, in a medical negligence case, the claimant is not given a copy of their own notes. Although the solicitor obtains full disclosure of the notes, on behalf of their client, it does not occur to them to show them to the client. It often falls to the expert (see below) to introduce the claimant to his/her records at the time of consultation.

## The consultation

It is essential, in my view, for the expert instructed on behalf of the surviving victim of a medical accident always to see the claimant. In the case of a baby damaged at the time of birth, the expert should see the mother and sometimes others present at the birth. While this is generally advisable, there are a number of instances where it is absolutely *indispensable*. Where the matter at issue is related to advice or consent, you cannot expect to appreciate the claimant's understanding of the advice given without an interview. Only the expert knows what options *might* have been put to the claimant, and such matters cannot be dealt with in a statement, however carefully composed by a non-medically trained solicitor.

In certain forms of birth injury, it is essential to know precisely what happened, matters that are often not revealed in the contemporary records. Thus, in shoulder dystocia, the mother and her birth partner often will have remembered important details that help the expert in the understanding of what was done in an attempt to relieve the dystocia. The hospital notes are often remarkably silent on these matters and everything will depend upon a clear reconstruction of the events surrounding birth.

Solicitors often question the need for the expert to see the claimant, and in my early career I had not learned this lesson and sometimes omitted this crucial step. In the past 25 years, I have made it an absolute rule and have never regretted it.

It will sometimes be clear to the claimant's expert that the claimant's own view of events is different from that revealed by the medical records. Here, the interview with the claimant (with all of the medical records available) takes on a particular significance. Often, with the aid of the medical records, the claimant's memory will be refreshed and he/she will realise that they are in error. Sometimes, the claimant is adamant that their version is correct and that the hospital records are wrong. It is not part of your duty to adjudicate between two versions of events. When it comes to recording events in the report, you must be careful to record both versions. It will be for a court to decide which version of events it accepts. Sometimes, you will be able to assist in explaining to the court why certain events could or could not have happened for purely medical/technical reasons. Only in that regard can the expert assist a court in deciding between opposing sets of facts.

In about half of the medical negligence cases referred to me by claimant solicitors, I am unable to support the claimant's case. It is particularly helpful, when writing a negative report, to have had the opportunity to see the claimant and perhaps explain some of the mysteries of the medical treatment which had so far eluded her. Claimants are much more likely to accept a negative expert report if they have had the opportunity of meeting the expert, giving their point of view and listening to the explanation of medical events.

In all personal injury cases, the particulars of claim must be accompanied by a report 'from a medical practitioner about the personal injuries [the claimant] alleges in his claim'(CPR16 PD 4.3). It is, of course, impossible to produce such a report without seeing the claimant. One might think that it was also difficult to produce a causation report without seeing the claimant, but I am surprised how often paediatric neurologists seek to do so, using only the medical notes as source material.

As a defendant expert, you will unfortunately seldom be offered the opportunity of first-hand discussion with the healthcare professionals associated with the accident – except perhaps at a later stage in conference.

# The report

## General

Part 35 of the CPR (Appendix 7.2) and the associated Practice Direction (PD; Appendix 7.3)[9] lay down clearly what is to be in the report. You must include a declaration that you understand your duty to the court and have complied with that duty; the report must contain a statement setting out the substance of all material instructions (whether written or oral). The statement should summarize the facts and instructions given to the expert which are 'material to the opinions expressed in the report...' (PD 1.2[8]). Only with experience will experts know how much detail the courts require, and there will probably be some variation.

The report must be verified by a statement of truth, the specific terms of which are laid out in the PD:

> *I believe that the facts I have stated in this report are true and that the opinions I have expressed are correct.*

The form of the declaration is not specified either in Part 35 or in the Practice Direction. It is for the expert to decide on the appropriate wording, but a model declaration has been produced by the Expert Witness Institute[*] (see Box 7.6).

Such a declaration and statement of truth is, of course, only relevant to a report which is intended for disclosure. Reports written only for advice must, of course, represent the expert's honest opinion but do not require the formality of a declaration.

Of particular relevance to medical experts is the requirement in the PD that the report must:

> ... where there is a range of opinion in the matters dealt with in the report –
> i) summarize the range of opinion, and
> ii) give reasons for his own opinion.

The court will need to examine the range of opinion, current within the profession at the relevant time, and will need to determine whether the defendant's actions complied with a responsible body of contemporary medical opinion, for that is the basis of the legal test of negligence. No expert should embark upon a report in a professional negligence case without a clear understanding of the law of negligence, clearly enunciated in the case of *Bolam v Friern HMC*:[16]

---

\* Expert Witness Institute, 8–16 Great New Street, London EC4 3BN

A doctor is not guilty of negligence if he has acted in accordance with the practice accepted as proper by a responsible body of medical men skilled in that particular art...

The principles were subsequently reiterated in the higher courts:

The concept of 'the responsible body of medical opinion' was first referred to and approved by the House of Lords in 1981[6] in a case about very different fact. That decision meant that, depending on the facts and circumstances of the individual case and the quality of the expert evidence given, the 'responsible body of medical opinion' concept became binding as a rule of evidence in courts in the UK. Further consideration was given in 1984.[17] The concept was extended by the House of Lords in the following year [18] concerning information to be provided to a patient to secure consent.[17]

---

**Box 7.6.** *Expert Witness Institute model of the declaration*

**Declaration**
1. I understand that my overriding duty is to the court, both in preparing reports and in giving oral evidence.
2. I have set out in my report what I understand from those instructing me to be the questions in respect of which my opinion as an expert are required.
3. I have done my best, in preparing this report, to be accurate and complete. I have mentioned all matters which I regard as relevant to the opinions I have expressed. All of the matters on which I have expressed an opinion lie within my field of expertise.
4. I have drawn to the attention of the court all matters, of which I am aware, which might adversely affect my opinion.
5. Wherever I have no personal knowledge, I have indicated the source of factual information.
6. I have not included anything in this report which has been suggested to me by anyone, including the lawyers instructing me, without forming my own independent view of the matter.
7. Where, in my view, there is a range of reasonable opinion, I have indicated the extent of that range in the report.
8. At the time of signing the report, I consider it to be complete and accurate. I will notify those instructing me if, for any reason, I subsequently consider that the report requires any correction or qualification.
9. I understand that this report will be the evidence that I will give under oath, subject to any correction or qualification I may make before swearing to its veracity.
10 I have attached to this report a summary of my instructions.

**I believe that the facts I have stated in this report are true and that the opinions I have expressed are correct.**

In a more recent case, the House of Lords[19] considered the matter again. In that case, Lord Browne-Wilkinson considered the application of the *Bolam* principle to the question of causation:

> His Lordship then said that in his view, a Court is not bound to hold that a defendant doctor escapes liability for negligent treatment or diagnosis just because he leads evidence from a number of medical experts genuinely of the opinion that the defendant's treatment or diagnosis accords with sound medical practice.[20]

Thus, in a professional negligence case the expert must not only explain what was done but also must assist the court to understand the range of medical opinion current at the time about what *should* have been done. The claimant expert must then justify his criticism by reference to the full range of responsible medical opinion.

## The first report

Whilst in a personal injury case a single report may suffice, in a medical negligence case the first report will be based on incomplete information in almost every case. It follows that the first report will rarely, in a medical negligence case, be appropriate for disclosure; nor will it form the basis of the expert's oral evidence. The purpose of the first report is to enable the lawyers of the party instructed (claimant or defendant) to assess the merits of the claim and to present the case to the court. Only at a later stage, when all of the factual evidence has been exchanged and the cases of both sides have been fully stated to the court, will it be possible for the expert to produce a report suitable for disclosure.

Thus, as the defendant expert, when first asked to report you will not have seen the claimant's witness statement although you should be provided with all of the pre-action correspondence and the statement of case. It is essential that you see not only the full medical records but also witness statements from every healthcare practitioner involved in the case. Your own investigation may well reveal the need for further witness evidence to be obtained.

When instructed for the claimant, you will have the first drafts of witness statements of the claimant and (where appropriate) friends and relatives, and will have all the relevant medical records. You will have, at the beginning, a somewhat 'one-eyed' view, for you will know (save only what is recorded in the medical records) nothing of what the defendant clinicians will say about their actions. Thus, the preliminary report, whether by claimant or defendant expert, is for the advice of solicitor and counsel in assessing the merits of the claim and in drafting the statement of case, or the defence to it. It will not be intended for disclosure to the court, for it will be based on an incomplete set of facts.

The format of the report is a matter of personal style, but certain basic principles must be observed. There are excellent publications explaining how a report should be written[21] and courses on report writing are run by the Expert Witness Institute and by Bond Solon*. These are highly recommended for the inexperienced.

The report should have a title page setting out clearly the identity of both the case and the instructing solicitors. It should contain the date and the name and address of the author. Neither a *curriculum vitae* of the author nor the declaration (with the statement of truth) is necessary for a first report, since it will not be disclosed. The report should have an index and either lines (preferably) or paragraphs should be numbered, for ease of reference both in conference and in court. The report should begin with a list of the documents seen and, if appropriate, the persons interviewed. Thereafter, the report resolves itself into three parts.

The first and largest part of the report consists of a careful analysis of all of the hospital records. With the aid of the records (and, for a claimant, the consultation), the expert reconstructs the events in a way which an intelligent educated lay person can understand. Although it is not essential to include all the details of the events of the case in the report, it is often helpful to the court to do so in a detailed and explicit form. Your ambition as the main liability expert on either side is that your report should stand alone and should provide an easy reference document for the judge, should the case come before a court. The reconstruction should contain relevant quotations from the notes, appropriately referred to the paginated bundle.

In the second part, the expert should go on to explain the technical matters involved. In a personal injury case, this may involve explanation of the injury and its affects on bodily function. In medical negligence, it will involve a full explanation of the disease process or injury and an account of the full range of medical opinion – *at the time* – concerning diagnosis and treatment. Some explanatory material in complex cases may, with benefit, be separated from the main narrative into an appendix.

The third part of the report should relate the case in point to this technical explanation. You should set out a critical appraisal of the standards of care, comparing them with the range of medical opinion current at the time. Finally, you should give an unequivocal assessment of the standards of care and, if you believe these to have been defective, should list the areas in which care fell

---

* Bond Solon, 11 Haymarket, London SW1Y 4BP.

short of the reasonable standard to be expected. In this discussion, you should avoid the use of the term 'negligence', since this is a question of law and may be misunderstood by doctors; in any event, it is for the court to decide after hearing evidence what is acceptable to the profession and hence whether the care has been negligent.

In forming this opinion, you should refer to standard textbooks, for they define what is an acceptable standard. Sometime, it is useful to refer to learned scientific papers, but they often reflect matters that are still under debate and on which there may well be more than one opinion. Such articles can be particularly useful to rebut the view that a particular practice is not acceptable, or conversely to establish that there is a responsible body of medical opinion of a contrary view. It is important that such references should antedate the incident. Where possible, the courts will be impressed by an evidence-based argument. Unfortunately, much of medical practice is still empirical and based on anecdote and textbook learning. Not all 'evidence-based medicine' represents ultimate truth, particularly if it runs contrary to common sense.

The report should end with a summary clearly stating the expert's opinion. Some experts put the summary at the beginning of the report. It is a matter of personal style; I prefer the summary to come at the end, so that the reader can understand how the opinions expressed in the summary have been arrived at.

## The covering letter

Your report should be accompanied by a covering letter. In the letter, it may be appropriate to give a simple overview of the report's contents and draw the attention of solicitors to further material required in order to refine the expert's opinion. Where additional experts are required, to cover areas that lie outside your expertise, solicitors will often be grateful for advice as to where to find a suitably trained and experienced colleague. Here, the expert is acting as adviser, not witness. Your duty here is to the client, for having given an opinion which supports the client's case, you have a duty to see that that opinion is expressed properly with appropriate support from experts in other fields.

There is no place in the covering letter for additional material that runs contrary to the opinion given in the report. It is not your role to leave out the uncomfortable parts of the factual evidence that might be inconvenient to the party who instructs you. As an expert, you must remember that your overriding duty is to the court, and your report therefore must contain *all* the relevant facts, not just those which happen to fit the party's case. You are also required (CPR35 PD1.2[5]), where there is a range of opinion, to summarize that range and give reasons for your own opinion; if there is a contrary view, it should be in the report, not in a covering letter.

## Conference

The earlier the expert is involved in a meeting with solicitor and counsel, the better. If possible, this should take place before any report is written; this will ensure that the expert's mind is directed to the legal issues, what has to be proved and where the other side will direct its attack. This will mean that counsel has a report with which to draft the statement of case with confidence and which there should be no need to amend later. Time spent in conference is well worth the expense as, in the long run, it saves both time and money. Neither the claimant nor the defendant can mount their cases properly without early and full consultation between the lawyers, the experts and the client (either patient or doctor). Here, again, the expert is acting as adviser, assisting the lawyers with explanation of technical material and assessment of the merits of the case.

Conference is a vital learning process for both lawyer and doctor. For the doctor, it provides an excellent opportunity to explain matters that, on paper, are often quite opaque. X-rays and other images viewed in conference will often become intelligible to the layman – both client and lawyer. Laying out several metres of CTG enables counsel to understand the document in a way that cannot be approached on paper. Orthopaedic models may be helpful in understanding complex anatomy. With the aid of a doll and pelvis, the mysteries of the mechanics of labour can be understood more easily. Conversely, it is often only in conference that the inexperienced expert understands the questions he is asked to address. Experienced counsel going through an expert's report methodically and critically can be a most rewarding (not to say chastening) experience. Much better for the expert to have errors pointed out to him in conference than discovered, rather too late, in the witness box.

## The statement of case

The statement of case is the formal statement of the claimant's case, answered by a defence. Neither document can sensibly be served without expert opinion, for it is upon the expert's evidence that the parties will need to rely in court to prove the case. If documents are exchanged which contain allegations (or defences) that you, as the expert, cannot support, there will have to be amendments later – or the case will be lost.

Once more, you are acting as adviser in assisting counsel in the drafting of the particulars of claim, or the defence to it, so that only those matters which you can support are pleaded. It may at a later time be necessary for the lawyers to produce amendments to the statement of case or further information, at the request of the other side. Here, too, your role as adviser is critical, and it is essential that you should see all those matters relating to your own expertise that are the subject of these documents.

## The final report

The purpose of the final report is that it forms the basis of the oral evidence that you will give to the court. The report should be addressed to the court and should be written with a full understanding of the expert's declaration and all that it implies.

Before you can finalize a report for disclosure, you will need to have before you *all* the factual evidence likely to be adduced at trial. You must therefore see all of the lay witness evidence to be called. By the time you are asked to produce such a report, each side's case will have been clarified in the exchange of court documents; and you will have had an opportunity to test your views in conference with solicitor and counsel. It may be entirely appropriate for counsel to advise you on the drafting of the final report. You must, however, take great care to ensure that you do not include anything in the report which has been suggested to you by anyone, including the lawyers instructing you, without forming an independent view of the matter. You must, above all, resist any request to remove from the report matters which are relevant and which remain your honest opinion but which do not fit with the client's case.

The tendency for counsel to exert undue influence on expert evidence was criticized by Lord Wilberforce in a medical negligence case:[6]

> While some degree of consultation between experts and legal advisers is entirely proper, it is necessary that expert evidence presented to the court should be, and should be seen to be, the independent product of the expert, uninfluenced as to form or content by the exigencies of litigation. To the extent that it is not, the evidence is likely to be not only incorrect but self defeating.

Lord Wilberforce's language was repeated by Cresswell J. in *The Ikarian Reefer*[7] and is now part of the received wisdom on expert evidence. Whilst it is clearly right that the expert evidence should be the independent product of the expert, it is surely putting it too strongly to suggest that neither the *form* nor the *content* should be influenced by the exigencies of litigation. But for the litigation, the report would not exist. The Practice Direction supplementing Part 35 of the CPR (*qv*) follows the sentiment of Lord Wilberforce and sets out in detail the form and content of an expert's report.

The final report, revised so as to take account of lay-witness evidence, should be accompanied by a full *curriculum vitae*, a declaration, as required by Part 35 of the Rules' and a statement of truth. You must also provide copies of any authorities upon which you seek to rely in support of your evidence. In providing textbook references, it is essential to include the title page and the date of publication. No permission is required for the reproduction of these documents and the normal copyright rules do *not* apply, provided that the document is intended for use in the courts.

Once the final report is submitted and has been disclosed to the other side, it is then produced to the court and must form the basis of any oral evidence you subsequently give. If, between the final report and the court hearing, anything material changes (such as new information or a change of expert view), it is your duty to inform the lawyers instructing you so that the court is not misled. The expert's overriding duty in giving evidence is to the court.

## Written questions to experts

The CPR 35.6 introduced a novel facility for each side to question, in writing, their opponents' expert evidence. Written questions can be put only once and must be put within 28 days of service of the expert report. No timescale is set down for the replies. If the expert fails to answer:

> ... the court may make one or both of the following orders in relation to the party who instructed the expert:
> (i)  that the party may not rely on the evidence of that expert; or
> (ii) that the party may not recover the fees and expenses of that expert from any other party.

## Experts' discussions

The provision for experts' discussions existed under the old Rules of the Supreme Court but, until the publication of *Access to Justice*, was seldom employed in medical negligence or other forms of personal injury litigation. Lord Woolf expressed the view that expert meetings should be the rule:

> Given the potential advantages and the flexibility of the possible arrangements, it is difficult to see why there should not be at least one experts' meeting in all cases where opposing experts are involved.[22]

The experience of those who have taken part in expert meetings is that they are usually productive and often definitive. My own experience is that they usually obviate a court hearing. Even if the experts' meeting does not resolve all of the differences between experts, the number of outstanding issues, to be determined by a court, will be greatly reduced, thus saving expense and court time. More often, the few issues remaining will enable the lawyers on both sides to determine the likely chances of success and lead to an agreed settlement.

The Practice Direction is silent upon experts' discussions but the Clinical Disputes Forum (CDF) has drawn up guidelines (see Appendix 7.1) for use in all forms of clinical disputes where experts' meetings are appropriate.

The key to the success of an experts' meeting is in the agenda, which is drafted by the claimant's lawyers and agreed by the defendants, and defines and limits the area of discussion. It consists of a series of questions, so worded as to direct the experts' minds to the legal and factual issues in the case. As far as possible, the questions should be framed so as to be answered with a 'yes' or 'no'. Open questions tend to lead to prolonged and pointless discussion. The purpose of the experts' meeting is that, having addressed all of the live issues in the case, the experts, before they leave the meeting, draft, agree and sign a document outlining the areas of agreement and disagreement. Where there is disagreement, the experts should indicate the reasons for the disagreements and the ways in which they might be narrowed further before the hearing.

Part 35 of the CPR refers to experts' discussions, rather than experts' meetings. Solicitors often suggest telephone discussions, rather than face-to-face meetings, on the grounds that they are easier to arrange and cheaper. The economy is usually false. Face-to-face meetings are much easier to handle, particularly if there are more than two experts involved. The creation of an agreed final document is simplified greatly by the experts being in the same room at the end of the discussion.

Where the discussions are ordered by a court, the final statement (CPR 35.12[3]) will be produced to the court, and the experts will have some difficulty in departing, at a later stage, from the views therein expressed. However, in other respects, the meeting is 'without prejudice'; that is to say that the discussions which lead to those conclusions 'shall not be referred to at the trial unless the parties agree' (35.12[4]). The final document is no more than a refinement of the experts' views, and as such, forms the basis of oral evidence to be given in court. It is not a resolution of the case and 'where experts reach agreement on an issue during their discussions, the agreement shall not bind the parties unless the parties expressly agree to be bound by the agreement' (35.12[5]).

# Preparation for trial

Immediately before trial, counsel on each side will produce a written skeleton argument for the court. It is important that insofar as that skeleton touches on technical issues, it should be vetted by the expert.

# Oral evidence

To the uninitiated, the giving of oral evidence may be a most daunting experience. The court, and particularly the witness box, are as unfamiliar to the doctor as the operating theatre is to a lawyer. It is essential for the new expert to familiarize him/herself with the layout of the court and the procedure of the trial well in advance of the first appearance in the witness box. The expert's final report will have been addressed to the court and the expert will know, long before appearing in court, whether the hearing is in the County Court or the High Court. In a County Court (where the lower-value claims are heard), the judge – of either gender – is referred to as 'your honour'. In the High Court, the address is 'my lord' or 'my lady'.

The trial begins with an opening speech by the claimant's counsel, setting out the allegations to be tried. It is a good general rule that all liability experts should hear the opening speech, but for the new expert it is *essential*. After counsel has 'opened' the case, the factual witnesses for the claimant are usually heard. Sometimes, a claimant's case is heard in full, with the factual witnesses followed by the expert witnesses, before any evidence is called by the defendants. That was the traditional way of hearing cases in the civil courts. More often in recent years, that order has been altered so that *all* the factual witnesses are heard first before any expert evidence is called. In any event, if, as expert witness, you sit in from the beginning of the case, you will have an opportunity to see the procedure for examination and cross-examination of witnesses before you take your turn in the witness box.

In the days immediately before trial, you should read again the essential court papers. The most important single precaution is to re-read the final report, which must form the basis of the evidence you give orally. Inevitably, minor (perhaps even major) errors will appear for the first time. This is the time to note them, for all is still not lost. Having re-read your own final report, you should read the final report of the experts for the other side, identifying the strengths and weaknesses of both cases. You should prepare yourself for the challenge of cross-examination and should, on re-reading both sides of the case, establish a point to which you may reasonably retreat when challenged. You should be clearly aware of the 'bottom line' beyond which you are not

---

**Box 7.7.** *Preparation for trial*

**General:**
- ▶ Find out the address of the court
- ▶ See the court
- ▶ Hear counsel's opening speech
- ▶ Listen to other witnesses.

**Personal:**
- ▶ Dress sensibly
- ▶ Be familiar with the court bundle
- ▶ Re-read your final report
- ▶ Re-read the opposing expert's final report
- ▶ Identify the strengths and weakness of the case.

---

prepared to retreat. Your views should, by now, have been thoroughly tested by counsel in conference so that you are fully aware of the arguments likely to be advanced by the other side and also are aware of the extent to which those arguments can be resisted.

It is essential that, before going into the witness box, you should have a personal 'court bundle' with which you are familiar so that, in the heat of examination and cross-examination, important references are readily to hand.

On first entering the witness box, you will be asked to swear an oath. Most judges require complete silence and attention in the court whilst the oath is being taken. Immediately after the oath, you will usually be asked to produce a *curriculum vitae* and perhaps to summarize it before the court. The *curriculum vitae* should emphasize those aspects of your own career that are relevant to the case in question. In a case involving a surgical procedure, it is helpful to tell the court how many such procedures you have personally conducted and over what period of time.

The first part of oral evidence – the *examination-in-chief* – is the easy bit. At this point, counsel introduces your final report. This is the opportunity, if last-minute errors have been spotted, to point them out to the court so as to deprive the opposing counsel of the opportunity to do so later. Examination-in-chief may provide the opportunity for you to go through the final report, explaining in as much detail as is necessary for the judge to understand the issues. If so, it provides an opportunity to explain the jargon. The pace at which the expert gives evidence should be determined by the judge. The evidence is for the judge and it matters little whether anybody else hears it; it is essential that the judge should not only hear it but have the opportunity to understand it at a speed commensurate with the judge's own requirements to note it. Judges will usually take down the critical part of the evidence in long hand. Some

---

**Box 7.8.** *Examination-in-chief*

---

This is the easy bit:
- ► Explain the jargon
- ► Take it slowly
- ► Address the judge
- ► Watch the judge's pen

---

judges restrict or exclude entirely oral evidence-in-chief – in which case, your evidence to the court will be that which you provided in the final written report

You should face the judge when giving your evidence, address him and watch what he does with his hands. Is he writing? If so, watch his pen and speak only as fast as the judge can write. If the judge is not writing, it suggests that the judge either knows what he is being told already or thinks it insufficiently important to write down.

Sometimes during examination-in-chief, the judge will himself ask a question. Judge's questions are usually of the greatest importance, for they indicate the way in which the judge is thinking and the areas where the judge feels the need for more explanation and verification. At the end of examination-in-chief, you will usually feel that you have persuaded the judge of the wisdom and veracity of your evidence and that all is going extremely well. It is only with cross-examination that the expert's evidence is called into question.

In cross-examination, opposing counsel will challenge your evidence. In this exercise, counsel will be assisted by his own experts, who will be sitting behind him and providing ammunition for the questions. The attack may take a number of forms, perhaps attempting to discredit your standing, undermining your status and experience, questioning the relevance of the authorities upon which you rely or just goading you into anger so as to provoke exaggeration and excess. The temptation is to engage in argument with opposing counsel, argument which may become heated and which may lead to indiscreet answers, giving the impression that you are partisan. You should always remember that it is only the judge whose opinion matters; defeating opposing counsel is not the object of the exercise.

Answers must be addressed to the judge. It is a useful discipline always to turn towards the judge before answering counsel's questions. If this produces a brief pause then so much the better. An answer given slowly after careful consideration is better than one offered hastily in anger or irritation. If the question does not permit the answer 'yes' or 'no', you should feel under no compulsion to give way to counsel's insistence that it should be so answered. An explanation to the judge that the question does not permit of a simple 'yes' or 'no' answer is acceptable. Questions in cross-examination will often contain several propositions, each one of which has to be considered separately. Whilst counsel may offer a complex question expecting a single answer, you should not be tempted into compliance. It is entirely proper under such circumstances to turn to the judge and explain that the question demands three separate answers and that you will give three separate answers. If the question contains an assumption which is not true, that too must be explained to the judge. It is by no means unusual to be asked a question of the type, 'Have you stopped beating your wife?' The false assumption should be addressed calmly and rejected. Sometimes, counsel will put hypothetical questions to you. You should make it clear that the hypothesis is understood but that it is only a hypothesis and it may be helpful after the answer to the question to add 'but that is not this case'.

Sometimes, counsel's challenge is appropriate and the expert must concede. It is important to concede gracefully and to accept where an alternative point of view might reasonably prevail. Obstinacy in the face of convincing argument will not impress the judge.

Finally, when cross-examination is finished, the expert and counsel will have an opportunity of re-examination. The purpose of re-examination is to recover ground lost in cross-examination and to clear up ambiguities and inconsistencies in the cross-examination answers. Sometimes, if the line of questioning in cross-examination has been somewhat misleading, a few simple questions in re-examination may restore the balance. If you have been seriously undermined by cross-examination, no amount of re-examination is likely to repair the damage. It is something of a relief after a long cross-examination to hear, 'No re-examination, my Lord,' but the expert never knows whether that is because he has conceded nothing (and therefore no ground is to be

---

**Box 7.9.** *Cross-examination*

**Remember:**
- ► Answer to the judge
- ► Do not carry on an argument with counsel
- ► Do not let him get under your skin
- ► Concede gracefully where appropriate.

**Do not:**
- ► Exaggerate

**Beware:**
- ► the hypothetical question
- ► the compound question
- ► the false assumption question.

recovered) or whether he has lost so much ground that counsel considers re-examination a waste of time.

Sometimes, at the very end of the expert's evidence the judge will ask questions. These questions are often the key to the case. They indicate the area in which the judge believes he needs to investigate. The answers assume considerable importance.

## Opposing experts

When the opposing experts are giving evidence, counsel will usually need skilled assistance in mounting a challenge and, during cross-examination, will need his own expert sitting in front or behind him so as to feed questions and challenge wrong answers. In fulfilling this function, you are again acting as adviser and fulfilling your duty to the party who instructed you.

## The expert on the fast track

Some personal injury claims may be tried on the fast track, if their value does not exceed £15 000 and if the issues therein are not complex. There is at present no expectation that medical negligence claims will be dealt with on the fast track, at least for the foreseeable future. Since, under the new Rules, costs must be proportional to the value of the claim, it is unlikely that more than a few hundred pounds will be available in a fast-track case for the cost of expert evidence. At present, there is no intention that experts should be called in person in fast-track cases, although the Rules do not specifically exclude it in exceptional circumstances:

> If the claim is on the fast track, the court will not direct an expert to attend the hearing unless it is necessary to do so in the interests of justice.
>
> **CPR 35.5(2)**

The idea that an expert, in a contested case, can write an opinion which cannot be tested by cross-examination is a little disconcerting, but this anxiety is perhaps somewhat reduced by the ability of the other party to put questions to the expert, a facility explained in Part 35.6.

## The single joint expert

Part 35.7 of the CPR envisages the use of a single joint expert (SJE): '... where two or more parties wish to submit expert evidence on a particular issue, the court may direct that the evidence on that issue is to be given by one expert only'. If the parties cannot agree, the court (35.7[3]) may intervene. However appointed, the SJE will be instructed by both sides (35.8). At present, there is expectation that the main liability experts in medical negligence cases will commonly be jointly appointed, but SJEs are already a reality in quantum and some subsidiary liability issues. For instance, in a cerebral palsy case it is now not uncommon for a single neuroradiologist to be jointly appointed by both sides to explain and interpret brain imaging to the court. The SJE was very much a feature of Lord Woolf's *Access to Justice*[23] and his expectation was that the single expert would save costs. In reality, costs will only be saved if the SJE is appointed in a non-contentious area, for if one or both sides wish to challenge the evidence of the expert, they will, of course, need to instruct their own expert, since counsel is unlikely to be able to cross-examine a medical expert effectively without skilled assistance.

Such experts must take care that their conduct is determined by the principles of fairness and transparency. Instructions must be given in writing and it is essential the SJE receives written instructions from *both* sides. It is not enough for one side to issue instructions and to inform the expert that they are jointly instructed. The expert requires, at the very least, a written acquiescence by the other party. Ideally, the expert should be appointed by a joint letter of instruction. If that is not possible, separate letters of instruction must be exchanged so that each side knows what the other side's instructions are. It follows, therefore, that as an SJE, you cannot accept instructions by telephone for they cannot effectively be shared. Every communication from the expert to one party must be copied to the other parties.

If, as an SJE, you are invited to attend a conference with counsel, the solicitor(s) for the other parties should be invited to attend that part of the conference which you, as the SJE, attends.

Part 35.8(5) provides that unless the court otherwise directs, the instructing parties are jointly and severally liable for the payment of the expert's fees and expenses. The prudent SJE discovers, in advance, exactly what arrangements are to be made for the payment of his fees so that he knows to which party he may look in the event of difficulty.

## Alternative dispute resolution

A number of alternatives to litigation are available for the resolution of clinical disputes. As far as I am aware, arbitration has not been employed in any form of personal injury in dispute resolution. A mediation pilot[24] was run by the Department of Health from April 1995, for a period of two years, in two health regions – Yorkshire and Oxford & Anglia. Although the programme was eventually rolled out to include the whole country, the take up was small. A report on that pilot is still awaited but will, I understand, reveal that no expert attended any of the mediation meetings. The role for the expert in mediation, at least at present, appears to be behind the scenes in the preparation of the case.

The commonest form of alternative dispute resolution is direct negotiation. In many small claims where the issues are straightforward, claims managers negotiate directly with the claimant or their legal advisers. The claims manager will almost always require an inhouse expert opinion before agreeing to settle even a small claim. Similarly, a potential claimant will be unwise to proceed without at least a preliminary expert view. In such cases, the reports must necessarily be brief and inexpensive. Small claims not negotiated successfully may be suitable for the small-claims procedure.[25]

## The role of the assessor

Both Part 35 of the CPR and the Practice Direction refer to assessors. They may be appointed 'to assist the court', but the rules are not at present clear as to exactly how they are to be used and when their use might be appropriate in a personal injury or medical negligence case. The assessor's reports are to be made available to both sides, and the report may be used by either party at trial (35.15[4]), but the assessor 'will not give oral evidence or be open to cross examination or questioning' (PD 6.4). Assessors will thus be in positions of considerable power and their introduction has been the subject of considerable apprehension. It has been suggested that where experts meet and cannot agree, the court may point an assessor to 'adjudicate'. This would seem to leave little room for the judge. Where the court would find such an assessor remains to be explained. Development of the role will be observed with considerable interest.

## Conclusion

Expert practice is changing rapidly under the CPR. The underlying principles – the overriding duty of the expert to the court and the proportionality of costs to the value of the claim – were set out clearly in *Access to Justice* and have been followed through.

This would suggest that experts will be poorer and more honest than before! Experts on both sides will be required to rehearse *all* of the facts in the case, even those which are unpalatable for those instructing him; experts on both sides will need to consider the full spectrum of responsible medical opinion, even when it does not accord with their own view.

This should lead to earlier identification of the real issues and to speedier and cheaper resolution of clinical disputes. It is important, however, to bear in mind that most expert evidence is written outside the context of the Rules. The full impact of the Rules will only be seen on those cases which come before the courts; in the majority, in which proceedings are never issued, expert evidence will remain unregulated. The hope is that the atmosphere created by the rules will nevertheless influence the culture of expert evidence and lead to the kind of integrity envisaged by Lord Woolf in *Access to Justice*.

# Appendix 7.1 Clinical Disputes Forum: Expert evidence

## 1. Purpose of the guidelines

To provide guidance for lawyers and experts to arrange discussions between the experts in clinical negligence cases within the ambit of Part 35.

## 2. Application of the guidelines

The court may direct a discussion between the experts in accordance with Part 35.12 of the Civil Procedure Rules (CPR); alternatively, there may be a discussion by consent between the parties. In each case, the guidelines apply.

## 3. Time for expert discussion

(1) The court has power to direct that a discussion be held at any stage of the proceedings. This will usually be after exchange of experts' reports.

(2) Discussions may take place by agreement at any time, including before proceedings are commenced, provided that the issues have been sufficiently identified to justify discussions.

## 4. Purpose of expert discussions

The purpose of expert discussion is to identify:
(1) the extent of the agreement between the experts;
(2) the points of disagreement and the reasons for disagreement;
(3) action, if any, which may be taken to resolve the outstanding points of disagreement;

(4) any further material questions not raised in the agenda and the extent to which those issues may be agreed.

## 5. Arrangements for expert discussions

(1)  The agenda:

There must be a detailed agenda. Unless the parties agree otherwise, the agenda should be prepared by the claimant's lawyers (with expert assistance) and supplemented by the defendants' lawyers, if so advised, and mutually agreed. The agenda should consist as far as possible of closed questions; that is, questions which can be answered 'yes' or 'no'. The questions should be stated clearly and relate directly to the legal and factual issues in the case.

(2) The nature of the discussion:

The discussion should take place face to face or by video link. Exceptionally, and having regard to proportionality, the discussion may take place by telephone. Save in exceptional circumstances these guidelines (and in particular paragraph 6 below) should apply whatever the form of the discussion.

It is usually advisable to have separate agenda and discussions between experts in different disciplines.

(3) The experts should be provided with the following documents before the discussion:

(a) The medical records.

(b) If proceedings have been issued, the statements of case, the claimant's chronology, the defendants' comments on the chronology, the witness statements and the experts' reports as exchanged.

(c) If proceedings have not been issued then the parties should agree a chronology and provide this to the experts with witness statements and such experts' opinion as has been exchanged.

(4) Unless the lawyers for all parties agree or the court orders otherwise, lawyers for all parties will attend the discussions of experts. If lawyers do attend such discussions, they should not normally intervene save to answer questions put to them by the experts or advise them on the law.

(5) Timing:

(a) A draft agenda should be served on the defendants' lawyers for comments 28 days before the agreed date for the expert discussion. The defendants should, within 14 days of receipt, agree the agenda or propose amendments.

(b) Seven days thereafter, the claimant's lawyers shall agree the agenda. If, in exceptional circumstances, agreement cannot be reached, the parties should apply to the court.

## 6. Conclusion of the discussion

(A) At the conclusion of a face-to-face discussion, a statement must be prepared setting out:

(1) a list of the agreed answers to the questions in the agenda;

(2) a list of the questions which have not been agreed;

(3) where possible, a summary of the reasons for non-agreement;

(4) an account of any agreed action which needs to be taken to resolve the outstanding questions in (2) above;

(5) a list of any further material questions identified by the experts, not in the agenda, and the extent to which they are agreed, or, alternatively, the action (if any) which needs to be taken to resolve these further outstanding questions.

Individual copies of this statement must be signed by all the experts before leaving any face-to-face meeting.

(B) Before the conclusion of a discussion at a distance, identical statements setting out all the information required in paragraph (A) above must be prepared and signed by each expert. Unaltered signed copies must be exchanged immediately.

## 7. The experts' duty is to the court and those instructing experts must not give, and no expert should accept, instructions not to agree any item on the agenda.

# Appendix 7.2 The Civil Procedure Rules

## Part 35: Experts and assessors

### Duty to restrict expert evidence

35.1 Expert evidence shall be restricted to that which is reasonably required to resolve the proceedings.

### Interpretation

35.2 A reference to an 'expert' in this Part is a reference to an expert who has been instructed to give or prepare evidence for the purpose of court proceedings.

## Experts – overriding duty to the court

35.3 (1) It is the duty of an expert to help the court on the matters within his expertise.

(2) This duty overrides any obligation to the person from whom he has received instructions or by whom he is paid.

## Court's power to restrict expert evidence

35.4 (1) No part may call an expert or put in evidence an expert's report without the court's permission.

(2) When a party applies for permission under this rule he must identify:

(a) the field in which he wishes to rely on expert evidence; and

(b) where practicable the expert in that field on whose evidence he wishes to rely.

(3) If permission is granted under this rule it shall be in relation only to the expert named or the field identified under paragraph (2).

(4) The court may limit the amount of the expert's fees and expenses that the party who wishes to rely on the expert may recover from any other party.

## General requirement for expert evidence to be given in a written report

35.5 (1) Expert evidence is to be given in a written report unless the court directs otherwise.

(2) If a claim is on the fast track, the court will not direct an expert to attend a hearing unless it is necessary to do so in the interests of justice.

## Written questions to experts

35.6 (1) A party may put to:

(a) an expert instructed by another party; or

(b) a single joint expert appointed under rule 35.7,

written questions about his report.

(2) Written questions under paragraph (1):

(a) may be put once only;

(b) must be put within 28 days of service of the expert's report; and

(c) must be for the purpose only of clarification of the report, unless in any case;

(i) the court gives permission; or

(ii) the other party agrees.

(3) An expert's answers to questions put in accordance with paragraph (1) shall be treated as part of the expert's report.

(4) Where –

(a) a party has put a written question to an expert instructed by another party in accordance with this rule; and

(b) the expert does not answer that question,

the court may make one or both of the following orders in relation to the party who instructed the expert:

(i) that the party may not rely on the evidence of that expert; or

(ii) that the party may not recover the fees and expenses of that expert from any other party.

## Court's power to direct that evidence is to be given by a single joint expert

35.7 (1) Where two or more parties wish to submit expert evidence on a particular issue, the court may direct that the evidence on that issue is given by one expert only.

(2) The parties wishing to submit the expert evidence are called 'the instructing parties'.

(3) Where the instructing parties cannot agree who should be the expert, the court may:

(a) select the expert from a list prepared or identified by the instructing parties; or

(b) direct that the expert be selected in such other manner as the court may direct.

## Instructions to a single joint expert

35.8 (1) Where the court gives a direction under rule 35.7 for a single joint expert to be used, each instructing party may give instructions to the expert.

(2) When an instructing party gives instructions to the expert he must, at the same time, send a copy of the instructions to the other instructing parties.

(3) The court may give directions about –

(a) the payment of the expert's fees and expenses; and

(b) any inspection, examination or experiments which the expert wishes to carry out.

(4) The court may, before an expert is instructed –

(a) limit the amount that can be paid by way of fees and expenses to the expert; and

(b) direct that the instructing parties pay that amount into court.

(5) Unless the court otherwise directs, the instructing parties are jointly and severally liable for the payment of the expert's fees and expenses.

## Power of court to direct a party to provide information

35.9 Where a party has access to information which is not reasonably available to the other party, the court may direct the party who has access to the information to:

(a) prepare and file a document recording the information; and

(b) serve a copy of that document on the other party.

## Contents of report

35.10 (1) An expert's report must comply with the requirements set out in the relevant practice direction.

(2) At the end of an expert's report, there must be a statement that:

(a) the expert understands his duty to the court; and

(b) he has complied with that duty.

(3) The expert's report must state the substance of all material instructions, whether written or oral, on the basis of which the report was written.

(4) The instructions referred to in paragraph (3) shall not be privileged against disclosure but the court will not, in relation to those instructions –

(a) order disclosure of any specific document; or

(b) permit any questioning in court, other than by the party who instructed the expert,

unless it is satisfied that there are reasonable grounds to consider the statement of instructions given under paragraph (3) to be inaccurate or incomplete.

## Use by one party of expert's report disclosed by another

35.11 Where a party has disclosed an expert's report, any party may use that expert's report as evidence at the trial.

## Discussions between experts

35.12 (1) The court may, at any stage, direct a discussion between experts for the purpose of requiring the experts to:

(a) identify the issues in the proceedings; and

(b) where possible, reach agreement on an issue.

(2) The court may specify the issues which the experts must discuss.

(3) The court may direct that following a discussion between the experts they must prepare a statement for the court showing:

(a) those issues on which they agree; and

(b) those issues on which they disagree and a summary of their reasons for disagreeing.

(4) The content of the discussion between the experts shall not be referred to at the trial unless the parties agree.

(5) Where experts reach agreement on an issue during their discussions, the agreement shall not bind the parties unless the parties expressly agree to be bound by the agreement.

## Consequence of failure to disclose expert's report

35.13 A party who fails to disclose an expert's report may not use the report at the trial or call the expert to give evidence orally unless the court gives permission.

## Expert's right to ask court for directions

35.14 (1) An expert may file a written request for directions to assist him in carrying out his function as an expert.

(2) An expert may request directions under paragraph (1) without giving notice to any party.

(3) The court, when it gives directions, may also direct that a party be served with –

> (a) a copy of the directions; and
>
> (b) a copy of the request for directions.

## Assessors

35.15 (1) This rule applies where the court appoints one or more persons (an 'assessor') under s. 70 of the Supreme Court Act 1981 (1981 c. 54) or s. 63 of the County Courts Act 1984 (1984 c. 28. Section 63 was amended by SI 1998/2940).

(2) The assessor shall assist the court in dealing with a matter in which the assessor has skill and experience.

(3) An assessor shall take such part in the proceedings as the court may direct and in particular the court may –

> (a) direct the assessor to prepare a report for the court on any matter at issue in the proceedings; and
>
> (b) direct the assessor to attend the whole or any part of the trial to advise the court on any such matter.

(4) If the assessor prepares a report for the court before the trial has begun –

> (a) the court will send a copy to each of the parties; and
>
> (b) the parties may use it at trial.

(5) The remuneration to be paid to the assessor for his services shall be determined by the court and shall form part of the costs of the proceedings.

(6) The court may order any party to deposit in the court office a specified sum in respect of the assessor's fees and, where it does so, the assessor will not be asked to act until the sum has been deposited.

(7) Paragraphs (5) and (6) do not apply where the remuneration of the assessor is to be paid out of money provided by Parliament.

# Appendix 7.3  Practice Direction: Experts and assessors

This Practice Direction supplements CPR Part 35. Part 35 is intended to limit the use of oral expert evidence to that which is reasonably required. In addition, where possible, matters requiring expert evidence should be dealt with by a single expert. Permission of the court is always required either to call an expert or to put an expert's report in evidence.

## Form and content of expert's reports

1.1 An expert's report should be addressed to the court and not to the party from whom the expert has received his instructions.

1.2 An expert's report must:
(1) give details of the expert's qualifications,
(2) give details of any literature or other material which the expert has relied on in making the report,
(3) say who carried out any test or experiment which the expert has used for the report and whether or not the test or experiment has been carried out under the expert's supervision,
(4) give the qualifications of the person who carried out any such test or experiment, and
(5) where there is a range of opinion on the matters dealt with in the report –
    (i) summarise the range of opinion, and
    (ii) give reasons for his own opinion,
(6) contain a summary of the conclusions reached,
(7) contain a statement that the expert understands his duty to the court and has complied with that duty (rule 35.10(2)), and
(8) contain a statement setting out the substance of all material instructions (whether written or oral). The statement should summarise the facts and instructions given to the expert which are material to the opinions expressed in the report or upon which those opinions are based (rule 35.10(3)).

1.3 An expert's report must be verified by a statement of truth as well as containing the statement required in paragraph 1.2 (7) and (8) above.

1.4 The form of the statement of truth is as follows:
'I believe that the facts I have stated in this report are true and that the opinions I have expressed are correct.'

1.5 Attention is drawn to rule 32.14 which sets out the consequences of verifying a document containing a false statement without an honest belief in its truth.
(For information about statements of truth see Part 22 and the practice direction which supplements it).

1.6 In addition, an expert's report should comply with the requirements of any approved expert's protocol.

## Information

2. Where the Court makes an order under rule 35.9 (i.e. where one party has access to information not reasonably available to the other party), the document to be prepared recording the information should set out sufficient details of any facts, tests or experiments which constitute the information to enable an assessment and understanding of the significance of the information to be made and obtained.

## Instructions

3. The instructions referred to in paragraph 1.2(8) will not be protected by privilege (see rule 35.10(4)). But cross-examination of the expert on the contents of his instructions will not be allowed unless the court permits it (or unless the party who gave the instructions consents to it). Before it gives permission the court must be satisfied that there are reasonable grounds to consider that the statement in the report of the substance of the instructions is inaccurate or incomplete. If the court is so satisfied, it will allow the cross-examination where it appears to be in the interests of justice to do so.

## Questions to experts

4.1 Questions asked for the purpose of clarifying the expert's report (see rule 35.6) should be put, in writing, to the expert not later than 28 days after receipt of the expert's report (see paragraphs 1.2 to 1.5 above as to verification).

4.2 Where a party sends a written question or questions direct to an expert and the other party is represented by solicitors, a copy of the questions should, at the same time, be sent to those solicitors.

## Single expert

5. Where the court has directed that the evidence on a particular issue is to be given by one expert only (rule 35.7) but there are a number of disciplines relevant to that issue, a leading expert in the dominant discipline should be identified as the single expert. He should prepare the general part of the report and be responsible for annexing or incorporating the contents of any reports from experts in other disciplines.

## Assessors

6.1 An assessor may be appointed to assist the court under rule 35.15. Not less than 21 days before making any such appointment, the court will notify each party in writing of the name of the proposed assessor, of the matter in respect of which the assistance of the assessor will be sought and of the qualifications of the assessor to give that assistance.

6.2 Where any person has been proposed for appointment as an assessor, objection to him, either personally or in respect of his qualification, may be taken by any party.

6.3 Any such objection must be made in writing and filed with the court within 7 days of receipt of the notification referred to in paragraph 6.1 and will be taken into account by the court deciding whether or not to make the appointment (s. 63(5) County Courts Act 1984).

6.4 Copies of any report prepared by the assessor will be sent to each of the parties but the assessor will not give oral evidence or be open to cross-examination or questioning.

## Editor's note

The Civil Procedure Rules can be assessed in their entirety on the Internet (www.open.gov.uk/lcd/).

## References

1. Pre-action Protocol for the resolution of clinical disputes. *Clinical Risk* 1998; 4(5): 139–144
2. Clements RV. Essentials of clinical risk management. In: C Vincent (ed.) *Clinical Risk Management*. London: BMJ Publishing Group, 1995: Chapter 18

3. Lindgren O, Secker-Walker J. Incident reporting systems: early warnings for the prevention and control of clinical negligence. In: C Vincent (ed.) *Clinical Risk Management*. London: BMJ Publishing Group, 1995: Chapter 20
4. Tapper C. Opinion. In: *Cross on Evidence*, 7th edn. Oxford: Butterworths, 1990: Chapter 13
5. Folkes *v* Chard [1782] 3 Doug. KP 157
6. Whitehouse *v* Jordan [1980] 1 All ER 650; [1981] 1 All ER 267
7. National Justice Companies Nadiera SA *v* Prudential Assurance Company Limited, *The Ikarian Reefer* [1993] 2 Lloyds Rep 68; 81–82 QVD; *The Times*, March 5 1993
8. *Access to Justice*. The Final Report by the Right Honourable The Lord Woolf, Master of the Rolls. July 1996, HMSO IV 13
9. Clements RV. The New Civil Procedure Rules: Part 35. *Clinical Risk* 1999; 5(3): 90–92, 93–96, 97–98
10. *Access to Justice*. The Final Report by the Right Honourable The Lord Woolf, Master of the Rolls. July 1996, HMSO III 13.54
11. Lugon M, Secker-Walker J. Editorial: Clinical governance. *Clinical Risk* 1999; 5(2): 39–40
12. *Access to Justice*. The Final Report by the Right Honourable The Lord Woolf, Master of the Rolls. July 1996 HMSO IV 15. 67
13. Whitfield A. Status of the expert in giving advice in preparing a report for the court. *Clinical Risk* 2001; 7: (2): 60–62
14. Waugh *v* British Railways Board [1980] AC 521; [1979] 3 WLR 150
15. Huntingford P. Obstetrics and gynaecology. In: MJ Powers, NH Harris (eds.) *Medical Negligence*, 1st edn. Oxford: Butterworths, 1990: 688
16. Bolam *v* Friern HMC [1957] 2 All ER 118
17. Maynard *v* West Midlands RHA [1984] 1 WLR 634
18. Sidaway *v* Board of Governors of Bethlem Hospital [1985] AC 871
19. Watt J. Leading Cases in Medical Negligence: Bolam *v* Friern HMC. *Clinical Risk* 1995; 1(2): 84–85
20. Watt J. Leading cases in medical negligence: Bolitho *v* City and Hackney Health Authority. *Clinical Risk* 1999; 5(1): 17–20
21. Bond C, Solon M, Harper P. *The Expert Witness in Court: A Practical Guide*. Shaw & Sons, 1997
22. Bolitho *v* City and Hackney Health Authority [1997] 4 All ER 771; [1997] 3 WLR 1151
23. *Access to Justice*. The Final Report by the Right Honourable The Lord Woolf, Master of the Rolls. July 1996, HMSO III 13.51
24. Simanowitz A. Medication in medical negligence. *Clinical Risk* 1998; 4(2): 63–65
25. Allen P. Small claims court and litigants in person. In: L Thomas, P McNeil (eds.) *The Medical Accidents Handbook. A Practical Guide for Patients and Their Advisers*. Chichester: John Wiley & Sons, 1998: Chapter 22

# ▶ Appendix 1: List of Bodies

| | |
|---|---|
| **Academy of Experts** | 2 South Square, Gray's Inn, London WC1R 5HT; www.academy-experts.org/ |
| **Advisory, Conciliation and Arbitration Service (ACAS)** | Brandon House, 180 Borough High Street, London SE1 1LW; www.acas.org.uk |
| **Bar Council** | 3 Bedford Row, London WC1R 4DB; www.barcouncil.org.uk/ |
| **British Medical Association (BMA)** | BMA House, Tavistock Square, London WC1H 9JP; web.bma.org.uk/homcpagc.nsf |
| **Council for Professions Supplementary to Medicine** | Park House, 184 Kennington Park Road, London SE11 4BU; www.cpsm.org.uk/ |
| **Council for the Registration of Forensic Practitioners (CRFP)** | Burlington House, Piccadilly, London W1V 0BN; www.crfp.org.uk |
| **Expert Witness Institute (EWI)** | Africa House, 64–78 Kingsway, London WC2B 6BG; www.EWI.org.uk |
| **General Medical Council (GMC)** | 178 Great Portland Street, London W1W 5JE; www.gmc-uk.org/ |
| **General Dental Council (GDC)** | 37 Wimpole Street, London W1G 8DQ; www.gdc-uk.org/ |

| | |
|---|---|
| **Law Society** | 113 Chancery Lane, London WC2A 1PL; www.lawsociety.org.uk/ |
| **Lord Chancellor's Department** | Selbourne House, 54–60 Victoria Street, London SW1E 6QW; www.open.gov.uk/lcd |
| **Medical and Dental Defence Union of Scotland (MDDUS)** | Mackintosh House, 120 Blythswood Street, Glasgow, G2 4EA; www.mddus.com |
| **Medical Defence Union (MDU)** | 230 Blackfriars Road London SE1 8PJ; www.the-mdu.com/ |
| **Medical Protection Society (MPS)** | 33 Cavendish Square, London W1G 0PS; www.mps.org.uk |
| **Medico-Legal Society** | Dr Jill Crombie Honorary Legal Secretary Medico-Legal Society C/o Hempsons, Solicitors 20 Embankment Place London WC2N 6NN; www.medico-legalsociety.org.uk |
| **Royal Society of Medicine** | 1 Wimpole Street, London W1G 0AE; www.rsm.ac.uk |
| **UK Central Council for Nursing, Midwifery and Health Visiting (UKCC)** | 23 Portland Place, London W1N 4JT; www.ukcc.org.uk/cms/content/home/ |

# ▶ Glossary of Legal Terms

**Civil Procedure Rules (CPR)**    Rules laid down in July 1999 to regulate procedure in civil cases. The Rules apply to High Court and County Court cases in England and Wales.

**Claim form**    Formerly known as a 'Writ', 'Statement of Claim' or 'Originating Application' until the introduction of the CPR. The form by which a case is initiated in the civil courts by the claimant *(q.v.)* Often accompanied by a 'Particulars of Claim', setting out the claim in further detail. Claims will be allocated by the court to one of three 'tracks' – the small claims track (for disputes of low financial value [up to £5000]; usually heard by a District Judge); the fast track (for relatively straight-forward disputes of medium financial value [£5000–£15,000]; usually heard by a Circuit Judge); or the multitrack (for lengthy or complicated disputes and those of high financial value [£15,000 and above; usually heard by a Circuit Judge).

**Claimant**    Person bringing a civil claim. Known as 'plaintiff' until the introduction of the CPR. (In Scotland, known as a 'pursuer'.)

**Common law**    English law applied by the courts but not fully prescribed by statute, derived from ancient usage and judicial decisions (Precedent, *q.v.*)

**Courts**    Places where justice is administered. Many different courts exist; the principle ones are summarized below:

| | |
|---|---|
| **Magistrate's Court** | Court with local jurisdiction over criminal and regulatory matters. All criminal cases start here; more serious ones are transferred ('committed') later to the Crown Court for trial or sentence. They also hear licensing and regulatory matters (eg breaches of environmental and planning regulations). All cases are heard by Magistrates (*q.v.*) |
| **Youth Courts** | Magistrate's Courts dealing with defendants under the age of 18. |
| **Family Proceedings Court** | Court with local jurisdiction over family matters. At the same level as Magistrate's Courts and usually in the same building. Hear some private family cases (eg private disputes between parents over residence and contact with children and domestic violence disputes), and some public family cases (eg local authority applications for care orders over children). All public cases start here; more serious/complicated ones are transferred later to the High Court. All cases are heard by Magistrates (*q.v.*) |
| **Crown Court** | Court with local criminal jurisdiction. Serious criminal cases are tried here, as well as some forms of appeal from Magistrate's Courts. Cases are heard by Circuit Judges, and in criminal trials there also will be a jury. In strict legal theory, there is only one Crown Court but it sits in many places. This is but one of many legal fictions. The Old Bailey is the central criminal court for London, but it hears (especially in the famous Court Number One) some of the major criminal trials from all around England. |
| **County Court** | Court with local civil and family jurisdiction. Most private civil disputes start here (eg landlord/tenant, contract, negligence disputes). Cases are heard by |

|  |  |
|---|---|
|  | District or Circuit Judges. Some private family disputes, including many over matrimonial finance, also are heard here. |
| **Court of Protection** | A court within the High Court that deals with the administration of the property and affairs of mentally incompetent persons (ie persons suffering under a disability). |
| **High Court (Queen's Bench Family and Chancery Divisions)** | The High Court in London sits in the Royal Courts of Justice in the Strand. The High Court also sits in 'District Registries' in other major cities (eg Leeds, Manchester, Birmingham). Some civil disputes are heard. The High Court will also hear some types of appeal from Magistrate's Courts, Family Proceedings and Crown and County Court decisions. *The Family Division* deals with family cases (it also has – in London – a 'Principle Registry', which is effectively at County Court level for family cases) *The Chancery Division* deals with a wide range of disputes, including some types of commercial disputes and those over trusts, land, wills, etc. *The Queen's Bench Division* deals with all other cases – for example, over disputed contracts, negligence, defamation and other torts, etc. *The Divisional Court of the Queen's Bench Division* hears judicial review (JR) cases involving challenges to the legality of decisions taken by public bodies or authorities (such as government ministers, local authorities, etc.) High Court judges may sit alone or in panels of two or three to hear JR cases. |
| **Court of Appeal** | Sits in the Royal Courts of Justice in London. Hears appeals from decisions of lower courts in civil, criminal and family |

cases. Does not make findings of fact or decide issues form scratch – its role is purely that of hearing appeals on legal points from decisions of inferior courts. Its decisions are binding on lower courts (see 'Precedent'). Court of Appeal judges hear cases usually in panels of three, with the majority decision being binding, and will not usually hear evidence, only legal argument. Some cases may be appealed, with leave, to the House of Lords.

**House of Lords**

Properly known as the Judicial Committee of the House of Lords. It sits in the House of Lords at Westminster, London. It is the highest court of appeal in the jurisdiction of England and Wales. Hears only a limited number of cases – usually those concerning a new point of law or a point of compelling public interest. Its decisions are binding on all other UK courts (see 'Precedent'). Like the Court of Appeal, it hears only legal argument on points of law – it does not make findings of fact or hear evidence. The only way of overturning a House of Lords decision is after a decision of the European Court of Justice or the European Court of Human Rights, or after Parliament passes new legislation. 'Law Lords' (correct title: Lords of Appeal in Ordinary) sit in a panel of five or seven to hear cases, with the majority decision being binding.

**Privy Council (Judicial Committee of the Privy Council)**

A court of equal rank to the House of Lords. Sits in the Privy Council Office in Whitehall, London. Judges may be Lords of Appeal in Ordinary or senior judges from Commonwealth jurisdictions. They hear, among other things, appeals from the General Medical Council and the General Dental Council professional conduct committees. They also hear appeals from various commonwealth jurisdictions. Its judgments take the form of advice to Her Majesty The Queen. The Judicial Committee may sit in panels of three or five judges.

**Supreme Court of Judicature**  A generic term for the Court of Appeal and the High Court.

**Employment Tribunals**  (Formerly known as 'Industrial Tribunals'.) Tribunals with local jurisdiction over disputes between employers and employees, usually over such matters as unfair dismissal, sex, race or disability discrimination, breach of employees' statutory rights, or redundancy. Has limited jurisdiction to hear disputes over breach of the employment contract. Usually consist of three members: a Chairman, who is legally qualified, and two lay members, one of whom will have an 'employee' (usually a trades union) background and the other an 'employer' background (usually management).

**Employment Appeal Tribunal (EAT)**  Hears appeals on points of law from the Employment Tribunals. Sits in London. Comprises three members: a High Court judge and two lay members, who will be people with considerable experience of sitting as lay members in employment tribunals. The most senior High Court judge sitting in the EAT is known as the President of the EAT. Appeals from these tribunals are to the Court of Appeal.

**Coroner's Court**  ('Sheriff's Courts' in Scotland). Hears cases in England and Wales involving violent and unnatural deaths or sudden deaths of which the cause is unknown. They also consider Treasure cases (formerly 'Treasure Trove'). The Coroner may sit alone or, in certain specified circumstances, with a jury.

**Crown indemnity**

A term in common (but incorrect) usage to describe the system by which civil claims for compensation involving employed staff in the hospital and community healthcare sectors of the NHS are managed and compensated by the NHS for negligent acts and omissions arising from the duties of their contract of employment. (See, also, the NHS Litigation Authority [NHSLA] and the Clinical Negligence Scheme for Trusts [CNST].) Note: independent contractors in the NHS (such as GPs) have to arrange their own indemnity provisions, usually through one of the medical protection and defence organizations. Also, employed staff are not covered for any work (eg 'Category 2' work) outside their contract of employment.

**Crown Prosecution Service (CPS)**

The statutory body that decides whether or not a prosecution for a criminal offence will proceed, and if so, conducts the prosecution case. Headed by the Director of Public Prosecution (DPP).

**Damages**

Financial compensation awarded by the civil courts to compensate in cases of tort or breach of contract; for example, in circumstances where there has been a breach of a duty of care (see below) that causes harm ('damage'), physical or psychological. Damages may be *general* (such as compensation for pain and suffering) or *special* (for quantifiable items such as medical fees, nursing care, loss of pension, etc.) Assessing damages is a specialist skill and there are many 'heads of damage' (ie categories of compensation) that can be awarded.

**Defamation**

A form of tort or civil wrong. A defamatory statement is one that tends to lower the esteem in which a person is regarded in the eyes of right-thinking people. It can be divided into *libel* (usually a written statement) and *slander* (usually a spoken statement). A defamatory statement renders a person liable to pay compensation to the injured party. It is one of the very few civil actions that may still be tried by a jury. There are special defences to an action of defamation. These include justification (ie that the statement is true), privilege (defamatory statements made in the course of proceedings in a court of law or Parliament are not actionable) and 'fair comment on a matter of public interest'. Defamation is not actionable in respect of statements made about someone who is dead – only in respect of the living. It may be morally reprehensible to 'speak ill of the dead' but it is not unlawful.

**Defendant**

(In Scotland, 'defender'.) The person(s)/bodies (eg NHS Trust) against whom an action is brought by a claimant (formerly plaintiff). Also a person against whom criminal proceedings are brought (also known as 'the accused').

**Duty of care**

All professional health personnel owe a duty of to their patients, to treat them in accordance with a reasonable standard of clinical practice. A duty of care may arise or be assumed in other instances; for example, a driver owes a duty of care to other road users, an employer owes a duty of care to his/her employees (ie to prevent them coming to harm in their work). Someone who performs first aid assumes a duty of care to the person whom they volunteer to assist. A breach of a duty of care is what gives rise to a claim of

|  | negligence. Compensation is payable if the breach of duty causes injury. |
|---|---|
| **Equity** | Now part of the general law (before the 19th century, it was a separate branch of law within different courts). The principles of equity are derived from concepts of fairness and justice administered on behalf of the monarch by the Lord Chancellor. |
| **Evidence (Rules of)** | The detailed legal rules about the way in which evidence might be allowed to be given in court. |
| **Fatal Accident Inquiry (FAI)** | The Scottish equivalent of an Inquest |
| **Forensic evidence** | Evidence given for the benefit of, or in, a court of law (from *forum*). |
| **Forensic Medical Examiner (FME)** | A medical practitioner (sometimes known as a 'police surgeon') with specialist skills and who may be called to attend and examine patients who have been detained by the police or certain other statutory body (eg HM Customs and Excise). |
| **Forensic medicine** | Medical advice and opinion used in connection with the courts. It includes that branch of medicine practised by FMEs and by other doctors who prepare reports in connection with litigation and for courts and tribunals and who appear there to give professional evidence of fact and expert opinions. |
| **Forensic pathology** | Pathology that is concerned with the detection of crime, ascertaining causes of death in suspicious circumstances and evidence in courts of law. Usually practised by specialist pathologists, some of whom might be recognized by the Home Office to be able to conduct postmortem examinations in cases of homicide, etc. |

| | |
|---|---|
| **Hearsay evidence** | Evidence not obtained with one's own senses (sight, smell, hearing, etc.) but from the senses of others (eg 'Alan told me that Susan hit her boyfriend', as distinct from 'I saw Susan hit her boyfriend'). |
| **Inquest** | Proceedings in a Coroner's Court in England and Wales. It leads to a conclusion of who the deceased was, how, when and where he/she came to his/her death and certain other particulars required to be registered (such as date of birth, address, etc.) Also makes findings about the ownership of Treasure. |

**Judges:**

| | |
|---|---|
| **Lord of Appeal in Ordinary ('Law Lord')** | Sits in the House of Lords Judicial Committee and in Privy Council. Known as Lord Brown addressed as 'My Lord' or 'My Lady'. |
| **Lord Justice of Appeal** | Court of Appeal judge, known as Lord Justice Green. Sits in the Court of Appeal. Addressed as 'My Lord' or 'My Lady'. |
| **High Court Judge** | Puisne Judge, sometimes referred to colloquially as a 'red judge', as they sit in red robes. Sits in the High Court. Known as 'Mr/Mrs Justice Black'. Addressed as 'My Lord' or 'My Lady'. (The High Court of Justice sits in three main divisions: the Chancery Division; the Family Division; and the Queen's Bench Division.) |
| **Circuit Judge** | Sits in Crown and County Courts hearing criminal, civil and family trials and some appeals from magistrates and district judges. Known as 'His/Her Honour Judge Purple'. Addressed as 'Your Honour' (except in the Old Bailey, where they are addressed as 'My Lord' or 'My Lady'). |
| **Recorder/Assistant Recorder** | The same as a Circuit Judge, except that he/she sits part time, the rest of the time |

being a professional barrister or solicitor in private practice. Known as 'Mr/Mrs Recorder Yellow'. Addressed as 'Your Honour'.

**District Judge**

Sits in the County Courts, hearing some civil and family trials and pre-trial procedural (interlocutory) hearings. Known as 'District Judge White'. Addressed as 'Sir' or 'Madam' (don't say 'Ma'am' or 'Mum').

**Deputy District Judge**

The same as a District Judge, except that he/she sits part time, the rest of the time being a professional solicitor (usually) or barrister (occasionally) in private practice. Known as 'Deputy District Judge Blue'. Addressed as 'Sir' or 'Madam'.

**Magistrate**

May be a stipendiary ('stipe' colloquially). Paid, professional legally trained person, usually full time. Stipendiaries are now usually called District Judges, somewhat confusingly, or lay (ie the same as Justices of the Peace' or 'Justices', usually not trained lawyers; usually part time and sit in 'benches' of three [the middle person usually being the most experienced and known as the 'Chairman'). Sits in the Magistrate's Court, Youth Court and Family Proceedings Court (FPC). Hears family trials and hearings (FPC), criminal trials and hearings (Magistrate's Court and Youth Court), licensing hearings (Magistrate's Court) and regulatory hearings (eg breach of environmental , planning regulations, etc.) Known as 'Mr/Mrs Magenta'. Addressed as 'Sir' or 'Madam' (only police officers and very old-fashioned advocates will ever use 'Your Worship(s)'.

**Chairman/Tribunal Member** Most tribunals, whether employment or any other sort, sits in panels of three members, but may sit as a chairman alone. The middle member is the chairman, who in many tribunals will be legally qualified, and in most is the *only* person to be legally qualified. Addressed as 'Sir' or 'Madam'.

**Coroner**

A judicial officer who presides over inquests in the coroners' courts of England and Wales, to inquire into deaths that are sudden, violent or of unknown medical cause. Coroners also deal with finds of Treasure, formerly known as 'Treasure Trove'. Coroners may be lawyers or medical practitioners; some are both. Scotland has a different system.

**Judicial review**

Legal remedy for wrongful exercise of administrative power or a review of a decision of a public body.

**Justice of the Peace**

An alternative term for 'Magistrate'.

**Lawyer**

Divided into two types: solicitors and barristers. Traditionally, solicitors have conducted non-litigious affairs for their lay clients and prepared cases for hearings. Barristers, meanwhile, have acted as advocates at court and other hearings, drafted 'pleadings' (ie documents required in litigation) and provided specialist advice in specific cases. These roles are now less demarcated – solicitors have rights of audience (allowing them to act as advocates) in many courts.

**Legal Aid**

State-funded financial assistance for legal proceedings. Generally available only for individuals and cases that meet funding criteria based on means and merit. Now known as *Community Legal Service Funding* (see 'Legal Services Commission').

**Legal professional privilege**

The rule that protects the secrecy of communications between a lawyer and

| | |
|---|---|
| | his/her client. (It is much stronger than medical confidentiality or that of the priest–penitent relationship.) |
| **Legal Services Commission** | Formerly known as the Legal Aid Board. The body through which the state funds access to justice. |
| **Letter of claim** | (See 'Claim form' above). |
| **Liability** | The condition of being answerable to a court for your acts or omissions. |
| **Liable** | Bound or obliged by law (including equity). |
| **Libel** | See 'defamation'. Libel is the *written* form of a defamatory statement, but it also includes defamatory statements made in the broadcast media of radio and television. Because the written word is more permanent than the spoken word, libel may 'sound heavily in damages' if the words impugn the integrity or competence of the person about whom they are written. |
| **Negligence** | Usually a civil wrong (a 'tort'). It is a failure to attain a reasonable standard of care that causes harm (damage). Someone found to have been 'negligent' may have to pay an award of compensation ('damages') and the legal costs of the other parties in the action. If a negligent act is 'gross' and results in death, the person responsible may be charged with the criminal offence of manslaughter ('gross negligence manslaughter'). |
| **Particulars of claim** | Formal statement of a claimant's case. |
| **Pleadings** | Collections of formal legal documents encapsulating an action. |
| **Police surgeon** | (See 'Forensic Medical Examiner'). |
| **Precedent** | The principle that decisions of higher courts are binding on lower courts. Once a |

court has reached a decision, it becomes binding on all lower courts that try similar facts. A precedent is not binding, however, if the facts can be 'distinguished' – a principle that can sometimes leads to some interesting 'legal gymnastics' in order to avoid an unwelcome outcome. Only the House of Lords can overrule its own decision; other courts must follow them unless and until they are overruled by a higher court.

**QC**

A barrister who has been 'promoted' by the HM The Queen on the advice of the Lord Chancellor to the rank of Queen's Counsel. Colloquially known as 'silks' and sometimes 'leaders'. Appointment to silk is traditionally made on Maundy Thursday, each year. About 10% 0f practising barristers are QCs.

**Quantum ('the amount')**

The financial value of a claim for compensation.

**Responsible medical officer (RMO)**

The registered medical practitioner who is responsible for the treatment of a patient liable to be detained compulsorily under the provisions of the Mental Health Act 1983. She/he is accountable to the managers of the institution in which the patient is detained. He/she is usually – but not necessarily – a consultant psychiatrist and need not necessarily be approved under section 12 of the Act.

**Single joint expert (SJE)**

An expert witness who will provide expert evidence on their area of professional expertise to the court. An SJE is appointed jointly by the parties to the litigation – a practice that has been encouraged by the introduction of the CPR in order to reduce legal costs and court time. Like all expert witnesses, the SJE has an overriding duty

|  | to the court, despite being appointed by the parties involved. |
|---|---|
| **Slander** | (See 'defamation'). Slander is defamation by the spoken word. The principles are similar to libel, although there are some important differences. Both are forms of the generic type of civil wrong known as 'defamation', which gives rise to civil liability compensated by damages. |
| **Standard of proof** | Degree of certainty to be achieved for an action to succeed. In civil cases, the standard is simply on the balance of probability (more likely than not). In criminal (and some other [eg GMC]) cases, the standard is the much higher one of being satisfied beyond reasonable doubt (or satisfied so that one is sure). |
| **Statement of case** | Term introduced by the CPR to replace 'Pleadings' (a collection of formal documents encapsulating an action). |
| **Statute Law** | Law which takes the form of an Act of Parliament (ie has been passed by both Houses of Parliament and approved by the Crown). One of two forms of legal authority in the UK jurisdiction, the other being judge-made, or common law (*q.v.*). The UK, unlike some other jurisdictions, does not have a code setting out its laws. |
| **Subpoena ad testificandum ('Come and testify')** | A Writ issued by a court or other authorized body requiring the attendance of a person at court, usually to give evidence, at a stated time and place, subject to penalty for non-compliance (a fine or imprisonment for contempt of court). |
| **Subpoena duces tecum ('Come and bring documents with you')** | An order of a court requiring a named person to attend, bringing with him/her documents specified in the order. (Quite often, the individual may avoid the need to |

| | attend court in person if he/she make available the required document.) |
|---|---|
| **Tort** | Civil wrongdoing, not including breach of contract. Examples include defamation, negligence, wrongful interference with goods or with the person. Torts give rise to claims in damages. |
| **Tribunal** | A body appointed and empowered to judge, adjudicate or arbitrate on a disputed question or matter, or determine claims and disputes. |
| **Ultra vires** | A term literally meaning 'beyond the powers', denoting that an official has acted outside his/her authority. Actions and decisions made by public bodies that are ultra vires may be challenged by way of a judicial review (*q.v., supra*). |

*The authors of this glossary acknowledge with grateful thanks the assistance in its preparation of Miss Suzanne Palmer BA(Oxon), Barrister-at-Law, of Field Court Chambers, Gray's Inn, London. Any errors or omissions are entirely the responsibility of the authors.*

# ► Index

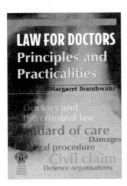